By the Editors of Consumer Guide

PRESCRIPTION
DRUGS
for People Over 50

with the Center for the Study of
Pharmacy & Therapeutics for the Elderly,
University of Maryland School of Pharmacy

Publications International, Ltd.

Louis Weber, C.E.O.
Publications International, Ltd.
7373 North Cicero Avenue
Lincolnwood, Illinois 60646

Permission is never granted for commercial purposes.

Manufactured in U.S.A.

8 7 6 5 4 3 2 1

ISBN: 0-7853-2465-8

Note: Neither Publications International, Ltd., nor the authors, consultants, editors, or publisher take responsibility for any possible consequences from any treatment, procedure, exercise, dietary modification, action, or application of medication or preparation by any person reading or following the information in this book. The publication of this book does not constitute the practice of medicine, and this book does not attempt to replace your physician or your pharmacist. Before undertaking any course of treatment, the authors, consultants, editors, and publisher advise the reader to check with a physician or other health care provider. Every effort has been made to ensure that the information in this book is accurate and current at the time of printing. However, new developments occur almost daily in drug research, and the editors, consultants, and publisher suggest that the reader consult a physician or pharmacist for the latest available data on specific products. All brand names of pharmaceuticals used in the text of this book are capitalized.

This publication was written and reviewed by members of the **Center for the Study of Pharmacy & Therapeutics for the Elderly** and faculty at the **University of Maryland School of Pharmacy.** The Center is a national model for pharmacy geriatric education and serves as the focal point of all geriatric education, service, and research activities within the school. The Center administers the Elder Health Program, a consumer drug education program for older adults. The primary goal of Elder Health is to ensure that patients understand and optimize their medication regimen by sharing responsibility with the health care provider for achieving desired outcomes.

Principal reviewer: Jean Dinwiddie, Pharm.D.

Contributing writers (drug profiles): **Aaron Burstein, Pharm.D.**, Assistant Professor, University of Maryland School of Pharmacy (UMSP); **Catherine Cooke, Pharm.D.**, Assistant Professor, UMSP; **Jean Dinwiddie, Pharm.D.**, Clinical Assistant Professor, UMSP, and Clinical Coordinator, Pharmacotherapy Clinic, South Baltimore Family Health Center; **Madeline Feinberg, Pharm.D.**, Clinical Assistant Professor and Director, Elder-Health Program, UMSP; **Lynn McPherson, Pharm.D.**, **C.D.E.**, **B.C.P.S.**, Assistant Professor, UMSP; **Becky Nagle, Pharm.D.**, Assistant Professor, UMSP

Contributing writer (introduction): **Rebecca Dougherty Williams** is a freelance writer specializing in health and medical topics. She holds a master's degree in journalism from the University of Maryland, College Park, and writes regularly for *FDA Consumer*, the magazine of the U.S. Food & Drug Administration.

Cover Photo: Picture Perfect

Contents

Introduction

Many adults over 50 lead active and independent lives, and they can expect to do so for many more years. On average, men and women today will live longer than any previous generation has, thanks in part to medical procedures and drugs that cure or manage diseases once considered fatal. Heart attack victims recover. Many cancers can be cured. Osteoporosis can be slowed.

Yet making decisions about medicines isn't always easy and clear-cut. When it comes to deciding what drugs work best for you, the best strategy is a team approach among patient, doctor, and pharmacist. Your doctor knows how to diagnose and treat problems. Your pharmacist knows medications, dosages, side effects, and interactions. But as a patient, it's up to you to be informed and knowledgeable about your medications and how they're affecting your body. This book can help in that task.

Prescription Drugs for People Over 50 is a complete guide to medications for mature adults. Even if you take no medications right now, chances are you will in the coming years. Or, you may be the primary caregiver for a loved one who needs assistance with his or her medication. If so, you know that all medications carry certain risks, especially for older adults. As a person ages, certain liver and kidney functions slow down and the stomach secretes less acid. An older person loses water and muscle tissue and gains more fat tissue, and aging produces subtle changes at the cellular level, too. All this affects how well the body absorbs, metabolizes, and eliminates a medication.

The more drugs you take, the more likely you are to have negative side effects from them. In general, older adults take more medications than any other age group— two-thirds of people over 65 take medications daily. People over 65 represent only 12 percent of the population, but they take over 30 percent of the prescription medicines and up to 40 percent of over-the-counter medicines.

All too often, older adults don't fully understand the instructions for their prescriptions. They may stop taking the drug after they feel better or because the side effects are unexpected or troublesome. Or they may forget a pill or two. Research indicates that about 40 percent of people using prescription drugs don't take their medications correctly. Each year, older Americans report more than 9 million adverse drug reactions, resulting in thousands of hospitalizations. To avoid such reactions, you should know what your drugs are designed to do, how they work, what side effects they cause, how they interact with each other, and how your body should feel when using them.

Prescription Drugs for People Over 50 provides up-to-date information on hundreds of the most commonly prescribed drugs, including what side effects you can expect and how serious they are, whether to take a drug with meals or on an empty stomach, whether the drug will affect your ability to drive a car, and whether a generic equivalent for the drug can save you money.

This book also contains general information on storing medications, instructions for using various types of drugs, how to read a prescription label, how to choose a pharmacist, and how to save money on your prescriptions.

Of course, this book is not a substitute for consulting your physician or pharmacist. Your doctor and pharmacist should be your first source of information on how to use a prescribed drug. Rather, this book is an accurate and quick home reference guide that offers information any time you need it. By staying informed, you'll be able to make choices to ensure that your years over 50 are as long, active, and healthy as possible.

TAKING MEDICATIONS SAFELY

Prescription medications can cure or manage many diseases if taken correctly. But taken incorrectly, they might cause more damage than if you had taken no drugs at all. Getting the right dose at the right time in the right way is crucial. This is especially true for older adults, who tend to be more sensitive to the effects of medication than other age groups.

Drugs come in many forms, from pills to creams. Many drugs come in more than one form. Each form of medication has a "delivery" method—the way it is administered. Some delivery methods may be very easy for you to master and some may not, depending on your own physical abilities and limitations. You may not be able to swallow large pills, or perhaps arthritis makes it difficult to put drops in your eyes. Tell your doctor or pharmacist what delivery methods are too awkward for you. There may be alternative medication.

Delivery methods

Liquids—Liquid medications are often taken orally. They are also used on the skin and in the eyes, ears, nose, and throat. Some liquids are "suspensions"; that is, the drug particles are "suspended," or float, throughout the liquid. It must be shaken each time you use it to get the drug particles evenly distributed.

If you're taking a liquid medication orally, be sure to measure it with a medicine-dosing spoon, not a teaspoon or tablespoon from your flatware at home. Home utensils range greatly in the amount of liquid they can hold. Your pharmacy has an assortment of medicine-dosing spoons. They are inexpensive and sometimes come free with a prescription. If a product comes with a certain dosing spoon or cup, it's best to use that one for that medication. Unless it is marked in milliliters (mL or ml) or in cubic centimeters (cm³ or cc), it should not be used to measure other liquid medicines.

Liquids or ointments for the skin should be applied with clean fingers, a small cotton ball, a cotton-tipped swab, or a small gauze pad. Don't use a large gauze pad because much of the medication will be absorbed into it. Never stick a swab or other object down into the bottle because you may contaminate the medication. Never cover the area an ointment or cream has been applied to with an "occlusive" dressing—one that does not allow air to pass through—unless specifically instructed to do so. For nitroglycerin ointments, measure an exact dose by squeezing along the measuring paper enclosed in the package. Spread it on your chest or upper arm in a thin, uniform layer at least 2 inches by 3 inches, and cover with the measuring paper provided. Use another site for the next application to avoid irritation.

Capsules, tablets, and oral powders—Most medications for adults come in pill form. A pill is designed to be absorbed into the blood stream through the intestines. Many people, however, have trouble swallowing pills, especially large ones. Pills can get stuck in the esophagus (the tube that goes from your mouth to your stomach) and begin to dissolve there. This can lead to irritation, chest pains, and vomiting.

Drink lots of water with each pill. Take a swallow of water before the pill, then wash it down with at least half a glass of water afterward. This will prevent stomach upset and help prevent toxic side effects from the medication. Don't take a pill lying down. Sit or stand up straight, and stay that way until you feel the pill go all the way down. If you feel the pill lodged in your esophagus, drink more water or eat some soft food such as pudding or a banana.

If you have trouble swallowing a pill, try placing it under your tongue and then swallowing normally after a gulp of water. You may also be able to break a tablet in half to make it easier to swallow, but check with your pharmacist first. If you still can't swallow it, you may be able to empty the capsule or crush the tablet into a spoon and mix it with applesauce, chocolate syrup, or some other small quantity of food. Don't mix it with a lot of food, or you might not get all of the medication down. However, be sure to ask your doctor or pharmacist if it's OK to crush the medication and mix it with food. Some pills are made less effective when mixed with food.

Others may have a special coating or a delayed-release action and can't be crushed because they lose their effectiveness or even become toxic.

Chewable tablets can be dissolved in water if you don't like their taste. Some medications come in a powder or pill form that must be mixed with liquids and then swallowed.

Other drugs, such as nitroglycerin tablets, are sublingual; they should be placed under the tongue and allowed to dissolve. They are absorbed through the lining of the mouth.

Drops—Ear-, eye-, and nose drops are all administered with a small dropper. Wash your hands before administering. Be sure not to touch the dropper to your eye, nose, or ear because the dropper can easily become contaminated and transfer germs back to the medication.

For eyedrops, wash your hands with soap and water. Lie down or tilt your head back. With one hand, pull your lower eyelid down gently, and place the drops between your lower eyelid and eyeball. For eye ointment, wash your hands with soap and water, and squeeze out a half-inch bead of the ointment in the same place. Close your eyes for one to two minutes, but don't rub them. Apply gentle pressure to the bridge of the nose and the corner of the eye so the medicine doesn't drain away through the tear duct. Try not to blink more often than usual, and don't close your eyes too tightly. Blot excess medication with a tissue. Wait ten minutes before applying the next drop; your eye can only hold one drop of medicine at a time.

Nose drops and sprays for congestion should be used sparingly and with caution. If you use some for longer than about three days, your nasal congestion will probably become worse than it would be otherwise. Other nose drops and sprays, such as steroids, must be used every day as prescribed to have an effect. Never keep a bottle of nose spray around after you have stopped using it because it may become contaminated. And never share any nose drops or sprays with another person.

Wash your hands with soap and water. Blow your nose before using nasal medication. For nose drops, lie down or tilt your head back. Squirt the proper number of drops into your nostrils. Stay in that position until you feel the medication spreading to your sinus passages.

When using a nose spray, sit upright with your head bent slightly forward. Squeeze the sprayer up into your nostril (without touching it to your nose). Keep squeezing the bottle until you take it out of your nostril, or you'll draw nasal mucus and bacteria down into the medication. After you have used a nose spray, lean your head back to allow the medicine to reach your sinuses.

For eardrops, warm the bottle with your hands (never use boiling water or a microwave). Wash your hands with soap and water. Shake the bottle before using it if so labeled. With the affected ear up, lie down or tilt your head to the side. Pull the top of your earlobe up and back with one hand to allow the medicine to reach your eardrum. Put the proper number of drops into your ear with the other hand, being careful not to touch the dropper to your ear. Stay in that position for a few moments until the drops move down into the ear canal.

Rectal suppositories—Rectal suppositories are used for a number of drugs, including laxatives, hemorrhoid treatments, anti-nausea medications, and even sleeping aids or tranquilizers. No matter their purpose, they're all inserted the same way. First, wash your hands and unwrap the suppository. Wear latex medical gloves if you are administering a suppository to someone else, or if you have long fingernails. If the suppository is at all soft, chill it in cold water a few minutes until it's firm. Coating it with petroleum jelly or mineral oil may make it easier to insert, but check with your doctor or pharmacist to make sure it is OK to do so. Lie on one side, and push the suppository (pointed end first) up into the rectum. If it comes back out, insert it higher, and hold the buttocks together for a few minutes to keep it in. Try not to have a bowel movement for at least an hour.

Vaginal creams, tablets, and suppositories—Wash your hands with soap and water. Before you insert any vaginal medication, read the directions. They may vary slightly between products. Some products contain an applicator to fill with medication, while others come with prefilled applicators. In either case, lie down on your back, draw your knees up toward your chest, and insert the applicator into the vagina as far as it will go comfortably. Push the applicator plunger to empty the cream, tablet, or suppository into the vagina. Always wash the applicator in warm soapy water afterward, and make sure it and your hands are clean before you begin the process. Often, creams are prescribed for infections because the patient has symptoms such as itching or burning outside the vagina. These creams are applied externally as well as internally.

Patches—Some drugs are absorbed through the skin using an adhesive patch. For example, nicotine patches help people stop smoking, nitroglycerin patches help prevent angina attacks, and clonidine patches treat high blood pressure. Follow the instructions in the package insert. Generally, patches are worn on a clean, dry, non-hairy site on the upper arm or torso (nitroglycerin patches do not necessarily have to go over the heart). Estrogen patches, however, are worn on the abdomen.

Wash your hands. Apply patches immediately after removing them from their wrappers. Hold the patch in place for about 10 seconds. Be sure the edges of the patch make good contact with the skin. Do not apply a patch to irritated or broken skin. Do not apply immediately after bathing; make sure the skin is completely dry. Change them as directed, alternating skin sites to prevent irritation.

Inhalants—A metered-dose inhaler (MDI) is useful for treating a variety of lung conditions. It consists of a canister (the medication bottle) and a holder with a short tube. The concept behind the MDI is that the patient inhales a cloud of drug. First, shake the canister well and then insert it into the holder. Hold the inhaler either right side up or upside down according to the specific instructions found on the package. Place the tip of the inhaler approximately 1 inch (2 finger widths) in front of your opened mouth. Without first taking in a deep breath, breathe out as completely as possible. In the middle of the next breath in, press down on the top of the inhaler until it releases the puff of medicine. Keep your tongue down to avoid blocking the mist. By starting to breath in before inhaling the drug, you are making sure that the medicine doesn't stay in your mouth but gets to your lungs where it is needed. Close your mouth and hold your breath for as long as possible (10 to 15 seconds). This helps the medicine reach all the tiny air sacs in your lungs. Breath out through your nose.

Rinse your mouth with warm water afterward to help prevent dryness. After using steroid inhalers, rinsing your mouth with warm water is especially important to prevent thrush—an overgrowth of fungus that can result from steroid use.

If you are having trouble coordinating your breathing and inhaling the medicine, an additional device called a spacer or extender is available with a prescription to ensure that you get the most from your MDI. These spacers are designed to attach to the inhaler and hold the cloud of drug particles for a few seconds. The patient breaths in from the spacer rather than from the inhaler. These few seconds make it possible to breath more slowly and help the drug to reach the base of the lungs. Spacers also allow the propellants in the spray to evaporate, making sure that the drug particles don't wind up on the back of your throat. If you notice any change in your voice after using an MDI, talk to your doctor about a spacer. Each brand of spacer is different; talk to your pharmacist about the proper use of the spacer with the MDI that you are using.

If you have more than one inhalant, be sure you know which one to use first. If you have any questions or uneasiness about using the inhalant, ask the pharmacist to demonstrate how to use it.

Over-the-counter medications

Over-the-counter (OTC) medications—those obtained without a prescription—provide relief for minor ailments such as aches and pains, colds and allergies, dry skin or eyes, and minor digestive troubles. While OTC drugs are generally safe, they all have side effects.

Studies estimate that older adults spend about one-third of their medication budgets on OTC products and that they tend to take about twice as many OTC drugs as prescription ones. The next time you go to the doctor, take a list of all the medications you use, including OTC medications. Ask your physician or pharmacist what kind of interactions might occur among the items on your list. Also ask your doctor or pharmacist if the recommended doses on the OTC package are right for you. You may be able to use half as much and still get the desired effect without as many side effects; you may be able to take more (equal to the prescription strength) and save money. Discuss any OTC purchase for yourself or any member of your family with your doctor or pharmacist.

Some common OTC products may cause problems when combined with your prescription drugs:

- Decongestants (in cold medications) can cause problems for those with high blood pressure (hypertension), thyroid problems, or diabetes.

- Antihistamines (in allergy medications) can cause side effects for those with prostate problems, or certain types of glaucoma.

- Aspirin can cause side effects for people with asthma, gout, ulcers, or bleeding disorders and for those who take blood-thinning medication, non-steroidal anti-inflammatory drugs, or diabetes drugs.

- Ibuprofen (as in the pain-relievers Motrin and Advil) can cause side effects in those with ulcers, kidney problems, or high blood pressure (hypertension), and fluid retention in those who take certain medications.

Storing medications

Most medications should be stored in a cool place with low humidity out of direct sunlight. A bathroom cabinet is not a good place to store medications because it is too hot and humid. A kitchen, bedroom, or hall cabinet is better.

If you have young children in your home or if they visit occasionally, don't leave your pills lying around on the kitchen table. Keep them in a cabinet with a plastic childproof lock securing the handles. The lock can easily be removed when children leave.

Don't keep medications by your bedside, either, where you may take them while you're sleepy and measure the wrong dose (one exception is nitroglycerin for those with angina). Don't set drugs on a window sill where the sunlight can degrade them. Don't transfer drugs to unlabeled bottles, or you might forget what's in them.

When your drugs have passed their expiration dates, flush them down the toilet or throw them out. Some out-of-date drugs are merely less effective, but others may be harmful. If you have a chronic condition for which you keep a large supply of medication, ask your pharmacist how long you can store those drugs safely.

When traveling, keep medication in your purse or a bag to carry with you at all times. Don't leave them in the car where outside temperatures can destroy them. For airline travel, carry your medication onboard in case your luggage gets lost or the plane is delayed and you can't get to your medication on time. Talk to your doctor or pharmacist about how to travel with medicines that require refrigeration. With some medicines, such as insulin, a few hours outside the refrigerator is not harmful, but others may break down or degrade in that time.

Special needs

Arthritis, poor eyesight, and memory lapses can make it difficult for some older adults to take their medications correctly. There are a few aids to make this task easier.

If arthritis makes if difficult to open child-resistant caps on medications, ask your pharmacist to put the drug in a bottle with an oversized, easy-to-open bottle. Large-type labels are not always available in pharmacies, but you can easily keep a magnifying glass in your medicine cabinet. Read the label under bright light.

Develop a system for remembering your drugs. The best system is one that becomes part of your daily habit. Some people use meals or bedtime to remember drugs. They reach for their medications each morning as they prepare breakfast and at night as they get ready for bed. Others use memory aids such as charts and calendar pill boxes. You can sort pills into separate cups for each part of the day, or you can even turn each medicine bottle upside down after taking a pill, and turn it right-side-up every night. Some people set the pills inside each bottle cap at night, putting the cap back on the bottle after taking the drug. Others set an alarm to remind them it's medicine time.

Those with serious memory impairments will need a family member or hired assistant to keep track of medications. Adult daycare, supervised living facilities, and home health nurses can provide assistance. An estimated 25 percent of all nursing home admissions are due to the inability to remember medication schedules.

It's always a good idea to keep a medication record card in your wallet or purse in case of emergency. A wrist or necklace medical tag is a good idea if you have critical health problems such as diabetes, heart disease, or severe allergies.

COPING WITH SIDE EFFECTS
Every drug has side effects. For older adults, however, side effects are often more severe than they are in younger adults. Sometimes even "mild" medications can trigger unexpected and uncomfortable symptoms.

How a drug affects an individual depends on a number of factors, including the patient's age, health, weight, metabolism, and whether he or she has any allergies or kidney or liver disease. Women tend to have more side effects than men. Sometimes side effects occur because of an overdose, while others are triggered by additional drugs or alcohol the patient has taken. Some occur as a result of the way a drug works in the body.

Older adults are more susceptible to side effects than younger adults are because their bodies metabolize or eliminate many drugs more slowly. With age, kidney functions and some liver functions slow down. Because of this slowing, older adults often need less of a medication to be effective, and a normal amount may cause unwanted side effects. Older adults may also be more prone to some medications because of subtle changes that take place at the cellular level.

Some common side effects of medications are confusion, tiredness, dizziness, constipation, stomach upset, sleep changes, diarrhea, incontinence, blurred vision, mood changes, and rashes.

Preventing side effects

Take as few drugs as possible—Not every ailment needs a drug to fix it. A change in diet or exercise may work as well as or better than a drug. For constipation, eat whole grains, fresh fruits, and vegetables, and drink lots of water (six to eight 8-ounce glasses daily). For mild osteoarthritis, you might be able to use heating pads or stretching exercises to ease stiffness and soreness. Ask your doctor, pharmacist, or physical therapist what non-drug therapies would be good for you.

Coordinate your drugs—If you have several different doctors, make sure each one knows what the other is prescribing. Ask for drugs that treat more than one condition. For example, your blood pressure medicine might also be good for your heart disease, eliminating the need for an additional pill. Always use the same pharmacy, especially if you are seeing different doctors. Then your entire prescription history will be in one place, and you can avoid duplications and interactions.

Know your body—Don't automatically attribute a new symptom to aging—it could be that the medication you're taking is causing an unwanted side effect. If you're sensitive to medication, you might need to try out a number of different medications to find one that's right for you.

Know your drugs—Make sure you understand what the medication is supposed to do, what side effects you can expect, which side effects are serious, how to store the medicine, what to do if you miss a dose, and how long you will need to take the medication. Make sure you understand *all* the explanations and instructions. Don't be embarrassed to ask questions. It is the duty of your health care provider to communicate in terms you can understand. Write down all your questions and don't leave the doctor's office or pharmacy until they are all addressed. If a question arises after your visit, telephone the doctor or pharmacist for answers.

Keep your doctor's appointments—By attending follow-up appointments, your physician will be able to evaluate your medication for unwanted side effects.

Ask for regular drug reviews—Whenever you visit your family or general practitioner, take all your prescriptions in a bag and ask that he or she review them. As drug experts, pharmacists can be an invaluable resource for medicine reviews.

Ask to eliminate drugs—Always ask the doctor, "When can I stop taking this drug?" and, "How do we know this drug is still working?" Sometimes physicians don't think to eliminate drugs as quickly as they think to add them to your regimen.

Use one pharmacist and ask questions—A good pharmacist will alert you to possible interactions between drugs, how to take medications properly, and whether there's a less expensive generic version of a drug available. Your pharmacist may also have more time to talk with you about your drugs than your doctor does, and it costs a lot less money.

Watch your diet—Food can have a direct impact on your medication. Some drugs are better absorbed with a fatty meal. Others lose effectiveness when taken with milk or high protein meals. Ask your pharmacist what foods you can take with each drug.

Follow directions—The timing of each drug is often important. "Four times a day" is not necessarily the same as "every six hours." It will be different for each medication. Ask your pharmacist to explain the timing of each drug. Read the label every time you take the medication to prevent mistakes.

Don't forget doses—Use a calendar, a pill box, or whatever system works for you to keep track of doses and get them right. The side effects may be less if you do, and the drug will be more effective.

Above all, be sure you understand your medication before you leave the pharmacy. Check your bottles and pills every time you leave the pharmacy, even if you've been taking the medication for years. If you don't know the answers to the following questions, find out from your pharmacist before you take the medication:

- What is the name of this drug, and what is it designed to do? Is this a generic or a name brand product?

- What is the dosing schedule, and how do I take it?

- What do I do if I forget a dose?

- What side effects should I expect?

- How long will I be on this drug?

- How should I store this drug?

- Should I take this on an empty stomach or with food? Is it safe to drink alcohol with this drug?

SAVING MONEY ON PRESCRIPTIONS
Most older adults pay for drugs out of pocket. Older adults also use more medications than any other age group, resulting in high pharmacy bills. You can save on medications in a number of ways:

- Buy in bulk. Many drugs are cheaper in quantities of 100. If you take a drug on an ongoing basis, stock up in large quantities. However, keep only as much of the medication as you can use before it passes its expiration date.

- When trying a new prescription, ask for samples. If samples are not available, ask the pharmacist to fill only one or two weeks of the medicine. Don't buy an expensive bottle of pills unless you're sure your body will tolerate them. Many pharmacies have free delivery services so that you won't need to make an extra trip if the new medicine does work out.

- Ask if senior citizens get a discount.

- Ask if a less expensive generic equivalent will work just as well. Many patients fear that a generic won't work as well as "the real thing." This is not true. Generics contain the exact same medicine as the brand name products, but are much cheaper because the generic companies don't have to pay for advertisement or for research and development of new drugs.

- Shop around. Call a few pharmacies to see what they charge for your medication. Be sure you tell the pharmacist the name of the medication, the strength required, and the quantity you want. If you find a drug cheaper somewhere else, your regular pharmacist might match the price if you ask. Don't be "penny wise and pound foolish," though, by spreading your prescriptions among pharmacies all over town. Using one pharmacy is still the best way to avoid duplications and inter-actions.

- Ask your doctor for free samples. Pharmaceutical companies give lots of samples to physicians to promote their drugs. Ask your doctor for some and you could walk away with a week's supply of drugs for free.

- For OTC products, ask your pharmacist for inex-pensive suggestions. He or she might recommend a discount product that works just as well as a more expensive one.

- Check medications available through the American Association for Retired Persons (AARP) and your local disease-related organizations (for diabetes or arthritis, for example). Let your regular pharmacist know if you obtain medicine from these sources so they can be added to your drug profile.

- Try mail order. For long-term drug therapy, you can save money by ordering through the mail. Use this service only if you know a drug will work for you, you need it on a continuing basis, and you can wait a few weeks for it to get to you. Again, compare prices before ordering anything. Only use a mail order service that allows toll-free telephone calls to the pharmacist.

CHOOSING A PHARMACIST

A knowledgeable and helpful pharmacist can provide valuable information to anyone taking medication. Most pharmacists don't examine patients, but they can act as medical consultants to evaluate drug interaction problems, side effects, and duplication of medications. Choose a pharmacist based on much the same criteria you would a physician: competence, service, convenience, and cost. Having all your prescriptions filled at one pharmacy means a centralized record of your medications exists no matter how many doctors you visit.

A pharmacist may either have a five-year bachelor of science degree in pharmacy (B.S.Phar.) or a six-year doctor of pharmacy degree (Pharm.D.). After an exam, they are licensed by their state's board of pharmacy.

Many pharmacies use technicians to help fill prescriptions. Some may have no formal pharmaceutical training, but every prescription they fill must be double-checked by a pharmacist. Some states allow more technicians per pharmacist than others.

When choosing a pharmacy, observe the way it operates. Is it clean and neat? Is it efficient? Can they find your order quickly, or do they seem disorganized? Is there a short or long wait for medicines? Does the pharmacy offer computer printouts with medicine information, and can the computer keep track of all the medications you take? Is the pharmacist available for private consultation? Does the pharmacist spend as much time with you as you need, or do you feel rushed out the door? Does the pharmacy have a free delivery service?

Large pharmacies often offer extended hours on weekends and even during the night. They carry many other household products, so one-stop shopping is easier. The drawback to a large pharmacy is that it will have a large staff, and you may never be served by the same pharmacist twice, or the staff may be too busy to talk with you about the special problems a medication poses.

A small pharmacy, however, is likely to have only one or two pharmacists on staff. They may get to know you individually, remember your special health needs, and alert you to potential problems with a given medication. They may also have more time to spend with you explaining how to take your medications. The drawback to a small pharmacy is that it is probably open only during regular business hours, and it may not stock non-medical items such as soap or razors.

Find a conveniently located pharmacy. If your drug store is located across the street from your doctor's office or near where you live, you'll fill your prescription more easily than if you had to drive a long distance. Some pharmacies have drive-through windows so you can stay in the car while waiting. And many pharmacies have free delivery, making location less important.

An important consideration in purchasing medicine is cost. If you have an insurance plan that is honored at a certain pharmacy, then going there will definitely save money. If you have no drug insurance or it covers a percentage of your drugs no matter where you shop, you may want to choose your pharmacist based on the cost of your drugs. Large pharmacies can usually offer lower prices than smaller pharmacies, but call around to check. Always balance the cost of the medicine with the availability of the pharmacist. Most experts recommend that you establish a relationship with your pharmacist just like you would with your doctor because all three of you are important members of your health care team.

READING A PRESCRIPTION LABEL
Reading a prescription is like deciphering code. Even if your doctor's handwriting is clear, the words he or she writes on a prescription pad may seem like gibberish. They are abbreviations of Latin and Greek words, a tradition from the days when doctors wrote everything in Latin.

Physicians use many of the following terms when writing prescriptions:

WHEN THE DOCTOR WRITES:	IT MEANS:	IT'S THE ABBREVIATION OF
aa	of each	ana (Greek)
ac	before meals	ante cibum (Latin)
AD	right ear	auris dextra (Latin)
AL	left ear	auris laeva (Latin)
AM	morning	ante meridiem (Latin)
AS	left ear	auris sinistra (Latin)
au	both ears	auris (Latin)
bid	twice a day	bis in die (Latin)
C	100	—
c	with	cum (Latin)
cap	capsule	—
cc or cm^3	cubic centimeter	—
disp	dispense	—
dtd#	give this number	dentur tales doses (Latin)
ea	each	—
ext	for external use	—
gtt	drops	guttae (Latin)
gt	drop	gutta (Latin)
h	hour	hora (Latin)
hs	at bedtime	hora somni (Latin)
M ft	make	misce fiat (Latin)
mitt#	give this number	mitte (Latin)
ml or mL	milliliter	—
O	pint	octarius (Latin)
OD	right eye	oculus dexter (Latin)
OL	left eye	oculus laevus (Latin)
OS	left eye	oculus sinister (Latin)
OU	each eye	oculus uterque (Latin)
pc	after meals	post cibum (Latin)
PM	evening	post meridiem (Latin)

WHEN THE DOCTOR WRITES:	IT MEANS:	IT'S THE ABBREVIATION OF
po	by mouth	per os (Latin)
prn	as needed	pro re nata (Latin)
q	every	quaqua (Latin)
qd	once a day; every day	quaqua die (Latin)
qid	four times a day	quarter in die (Latin)
qod	every other day	—
s	without	sine (Latin)
sig	label as follows	signa (Latin)
sl	under the tongue	sub lingua (Latin)
SOB	shortness of breath	—
sol	solution	—
ss	half unit	semis (Latin)
stat	at once; first dose	statim (Latin)
susp	suspension	—
tab	tablet	—
tid	three times a day	ter in die (Latin)
top	apply topically	—
ung or ungt	ointment	unguentum (Latin)
UT	under the tongue	—
ut dict or UD	as directed	ut dictum (Latin)

Instead of trying to understand all the Latin words, however, ask your doctor to explain what the prescription says. Over-the-counter medications have important instructions on their labels as well. Read these carefully before taking the product, and ask your pharmacist if a product is OK for you to use given your medical conditions and the other medications you take.

USING THIS BOOK

There are several ways to find information in this book. The drug profiles are listed in alphabetical order by generic name. Use the Brand Names Index (page 549) or the Canadian Brand Names Index (page 563) to find the generic name of the drug you want to look up, or refer to the General Index to find the page number.

There are several things to keep in mind when reading a profile. First, this book should never supersede your doctor or pharmacist's instructions. Under "Administration," you'll find instructions on how the drug is *usually* prescribed and taken. However, your doctor or pharmacist may have very different instructions. *Always follow your doctor or pharmacist's instructions.*

Second, under "Precautions," you'll find situations that warrant talking to your doctor about your treatment. These are not the only situations in which you should raise questions. Tell your doctor or pharmacist about *all* your health problems, medications, and concerns before you start taking a medication. Remember, during long-term therapy, new concerns may arise; *talk to your doctor or pharmacist whenever you have questions.*

Finally, under the heading "Side Effects," you'll find two categories: *Major* and *Minor.* If you experience any of the major side effects listed, seek medical attention immediately. These symptoms are often signs of allergic reactions or serious interactions that can be dangerous or fatal. The symptoms listed as minor, on the other hand, are mostly harmless. Although these usually do not require medical attention, you should talk to your doctor or pharmacist if they become particularly bothersome.

acarbose

Brand Name: Precose (Bayer)

Generic Available: no

Type of Drug: hormone (antidiabetic)

Used for: Lowering blood glucose levels in the treatment of non–insulin-dependent (type II) diabetes.

How This Medication Works: Inhibits the enzyme alpha-glucosidase, delaying absorption of carbohydrates from the small intestine.

Dosage Form and Strength: tablets (50 mg, 100 mg)

Storage:
- room temperature
- tightly closed
- protected from humidity

Administration:
- Usually taken 3 times daily with the first bite of a meal.
- Dosage is determined by your response to the medication and your tolerance of the side effects, but total dosage should not exceed 100 mg 3 times daily.

Precautions:
Do not use if:
- you are allergic to acarbose.
- medicine is beyond the expiration date.

Talk to your doctor if:
- you are on medication containing digestive enzymes such as pancrelipase or pancreatin.
- you are taking other oral diabetes medications such as glyburide or glipizide.
- you have liver disease, inflammatory bowel disease, ulcerative colitis, Crohn disease, or kidney disease.
- you have ever had hepatitis or an intestinal obstruction.

Side Effects:
Major: none
Minor:
- flatulence
- abdominal cramps
- diarrhea

Time Required for Drug to Take Effect:
Begins to work with the first dose, but it takes some time to establish the proper dose to control your diabetes.

Symptoms of Overdose:
- temporary increase in minor side effects

Special Notes:
- When you begin acarbose therapy, check your blood glucose level 1 hour after meals.
- Acarbose alone will not cause low blood sugar (hypoglycemia).
- Side effects generally decrease over time as your body becomes accustomed to the drug.
- Do not drink alcohol while taking this medicine.

- Do not discontinue this medication without checking with your doctor.
- It is important to take this medication every day, especially on days that you are not feeling well. Talk to your doctor or diabetes educator about how to handle sick days.

acetazolamide

Brand Names:
Diamox (Lederle)
Dazamide (Major)

Generic Available: yes

Type of Drug: diuretic

Used for: Treatment of chronic simple glaucoma and mountain sickness, and lowering intraocular pressure during and after eye surgery.

How This Medication Works: Decreases the rate of formation of aqueous humor (the fluid in the eye) and increases the kidney's excretion of sodium, potassium, bicarbonate, and water.

Dosage Form and Strength:
- tablets (125 mg, 250 mg)
- sustained-release capsules (500 mg)

Storage:
- room temperature
- tightly closed
- protected from humidity

Administration:
- Swallow sustained-release capsules whole; do not crush or chew.
- Take with orange juice or a banana to replace the potassium that may be excreted.
- Take with food or milk if stomach upset occurs.

Precautions:
Do not use if:
- you are allergic to acetazolamide or other sulfa drugs such as tolazamide, glipizide, glyburide, hydrochlorothiazide, chlorthalidone, metolazone, furosemide, bumetanide, or sulfamethoxazole.

Talk to your doctor if:
- you have liver disease, kidney disease, asthma, chronic bronchitis, or emphysema.
- you are taking digoxin, steroids (such as pred-nisone or methylprednisolone), cyclosporine, primidone, aspirin, salicylates, or diflunisal.

Side Effects:
Major:
- sore throat and fever
- unusual bleeding or unexplained bruising
- tingling, burning sensation, tremors, or "pins and needles" in hands or feet
- flank or loin pain
- skin rash
- unexplained, prolonged general tiredness
- convulsions

Minor:
- nausea and vomiting
- drowsiness or dizziness

- headache
- ringing or buzzing in the ears (tinnitus)

Time Required for Drug to Take Effect:
Tablets begin to work within 1 hour and continue to lower intraocular pressure for 8 to 12 hours. Sustained-release capsules begin to lower pressure in about 2 hours and continue to work for 18 to 24 hours.

Symptoms of Overdose:
- drowsiness or dizziness
- loss of appetite
- nausea and vomiting
- inability to coordinate movement
- tremors
- ringing or buzzing in the ears (tinnitus)
- numbness or tingling in the arms and legs

Special Notes:
- Drink 6 to 8 full glasses of water every day to avoid dehydration (unless otherwise instructed by your doctor).
- Use a sunblock with at least SPF 15 when outside because acetazolamide may increase your sensitivity to the sun.
- If you experience dryness of the mouth, try sugarless candy or gum, ice chips, or a saliva substitute.

acyclovir

Brand Name: Zovirax (Glaxo Wellcome)

Generic Available: no

Type of Drug: antiviral

Used For: Treatment of infections caused by viruses, including herpes simplex, herpes zoster (shingles), and varicella zoster (chicken pox).

How this Medication Works: Inhibits the virus's ability to replicate.

Dosage Form and Strength:
- tablets (400 mg, 800 mg)
- capsules (200 mg)
- suspension (200 mg/5 mL)

Storage:
- room temperature
- tightly closed
- protected from humidity

Administration:
- Dosage will vary from 800 mg 5 times daily for acute shingles attack to 400 mg 2 times daily as suppressive therapy.
- Take each dose with a full glass of water.
- Shake suspension well before measuring dose.
- Take until completely gone, even if symptoms improve.

Precautions:
Do not use if:
- you are allergic to acyclovir.
- medicine is beyond the expiration date or unusual in appearance.

Talk to your doctor if:
- you are taking probenecid or zidovudine.
- you have kidney disease.

Side Effects:

Major:
- skin rash
- swollen glands in the groin
- numbness or tingling in the arms or legs

Minor:
- nausea
- vomiting
- diarrhea
- loss of appetite

Time Required for Drug to Take Effect: May take several days to have full effect.

Symptoms of Overdose:
- kidney failure

Special Notes:
- Do not use for infections other than the one for which it was prescribed.
- Acyclovir is most useful for shingles if used within the first 48 hours of an acute attack.

albuterol

Brand Names:

Proventil Repetabs
  (Schering)

Proventil (Schering)
Ventolin (Glaxo Wellcome)

Generic Available: yes

Type of Drug: bronchodilator

Used for: Treatment of asthma, emphysema, and chronic bronchitis.

How This Medication Works: Causes the passageways in the lungs to dilate.

Dosage Form and Strength:
- tablets (2 mg, 4 mg)
- syrup (2 mg/5 mL)
- inhaler (90 µg/inhalation)

Storage:
- room temperature
- protected from humidity

Administration:
- When using the inhaler, allow at least 2 minutes between inhalations (puffs).
- If you have more than one inhaler, it is important to administer your inhalers in the correct order. If you are using albuterol and another inhaler, use the albuterol first. Wait at least 5 minutes before inhaling the second medication.
- Have your doctor or pharmacist demonstrate the proper procedure for using it and make sure they have you practice your technique in front of them.

Precautions:
Do not use if:
- you are allergic to albuterol, epinephrine, metaproterenol, salmeterol, or terbutaline.

Talk to your doctor if:
- you have diabetes, heart disease, high blood pressure (hypertension), problems with circulation or blood vessels, seizures, convulsions, or thyroid disease.
- you are taking any other medications, especially medications for heart disease, high blood pressure (hypertension), migraine headaches, or depression.

Side Effects:

Major:
- skin rash, itching, or hives
- difficulty breathing
- increased wheezing
- bluish coloring of skin
- swelling of face, lips, or eyelids
- fainting or dizziness
- chest discomfort or pressure
- irregular heartbeat
- numbness or tingling in hands or feet
- hallucinations

Minor:
- nervousness
- tremor or trembling
- coughing
- dryness or irritation of mouth or throat
- unpleasant taste
- flushing or redness of face
- headache
- increased sweating
- increase in blood pressure
- muscle cramps or twitching

- nausea or vomiting
- trouble sleeping
- drowsiness

Time Required for Drug to Take Effect:
Inhaled medications start to work within 60 seconds. Tablets take about 2 to 3 hours.

Symptoms of Overdose:
- chest discomfort or pressure
- chills or fever
- seizures or convulsions
- irregular heartbeat
- severe nausea or vomiting
- severe difficulty breathing
- severe tremor or trembling
- blurred vision
- unusual paleness and coldness of skin

Special Notes:
- If you are using albuterol as treatment for acute attacks, or to prevent exercise-induced asthma, it is important to carry your albuterol inhaler with you at all times.
- Sometimes a spacer device is used with your inhaler. A spacer device helps the medication get to the lungs instead of the mouth or throat.
- Check with your physician or pharmacist before using any over-the-counter medications.
- Save the applicator from your inhaler. There may be refills that fit into your applicator.
- Keep track of how many inhalations are left and get your medication refilled about 1 week before you expect to run out.

alendronate

Brand Name: Fosamax (Merck)

Generic Available: no

Type of Drug: miscellaneous

Used for: Treatment of Paget disease of the bone and prevention of bone loss in osteoporosis.

How This Medication Works: Reduces the rate of bone loss (reabsorption), making bones stronger.

Dosage Form and Strength: tablets (10 mg, 40 mg)

Storage:
- room temperature
- tightly closed
- protected from light

Administration:
- Usually 10 mg daily for osteoporosis.
- Usually 40 mg daily for 6 months for Paget disease.
- Take in the morning with an 8-ounce glass of water at least ½ hour before food, beverages, or other medication.

Precautions:
Do not use if:
- you have had a severe allergic reaction to alendronate or etidronate.
- you have severe kidney disease.
- you have low calcium levels (hypocalcemia).

Talk to your doctor if:
- you have kidney disease or ulcers.
- you are taking any other medication, especially calcium supplements.

Side Effects:

Major:
- low calcium levels (hypocalcemia)
- low phosphate levels (hypophosphatemia)

Minor:
- temporary increase in bone pain
- constipation or diarrhea
- headache
- muscle pain
- stomach pain

Time Required for Drug to Take Effect: In
Paget disease, 3 to 6 months; in osteoporosis, 3 to 6 weeks.

Symptoms of Overdose: Not known

Special Notes:
- Follow any diet your doctor has given you.
- If you are told to take calcium, take it at least 2 hours after alendronate.
- Blood tests are often necessary to make sure you do not develop side effects.

allopurinol

Brand Name: Zyloprim (Burroughs Wellcome)

Generic Available: yes

Type of Drug: antigout

Used for: Treatment of gout.

How This Medication Works: Inhibits the formation of uric acid.

Dosage Form and Strength: tablets (100 mg, 300 mg)

Storage:
- tightly closed
- protected from humidity

Administration:
- Only for prevention of gout attacks, not for acute attacks, which it may actually worsen.
- Drink a minimum of 10 to 12 eight-ounce glasses of water daily while taking allopurinol (unless otherwise instructed).
- Take with food or milk if medication causes stomach upset.
- Often, your doctor will start with lower doses of allopurinol and increase the dose slowly to minimize side effects.

Precautions:

Do not use if:
- you are allergic to allopurinol.

Talk to your doctor if:
- you have diabetes, high blood pressure (hypertension), or kidney disease.
- you are taking any other medications, especially anticoagulants (such as warfarin), azathioprine, or mercaptopurine.

Side Effects:
Major:
- skin rash, hives, or itching
- sores on mouth or lips
- blood in urine or stool
- fever or sore throat
- nausea or vomiting
- muscle aches
- difficult or painful urination
- difficulty breathing
- swelling
- unusual bleeding or bruising
- weight gain
- yellow eyes or skin (jaundice)

Minor:
- loosening of fingernails
- numbness or tingling in hands or feet
- diarrhea
- drowsiness
- headache
- nausea
- hair loss

Time Required for Drug to Take Effect: Starts
to work within 1 to 2 hours, but it usually takes 1 to
3 weeks to see the full effect.

Symptoms of Overdose: No specific symptoms
have been associated with overdose.

Special Notes:
- You will be required to have blood tests to determine the amount of uric acid in your blood.

- Check with your physician or pharmacist before using any over-the-counter medications.
- This medication may cause drowsiness. Use caution when operating a motor vehicle or operating dangerous machinery.
- Do not drink alcohol while taking this medication.
- Avoid taking too much vitamin C. It may increase the risk for kidney stones while taking allopurinol.

alprazolam

Brand Name: Xanax (Upjohn)

Generic Available: yes

Type of Drug: antianxiety

Used for: Treatment of anxiety, panic disorders, post-traumatic stress syndrome.

How This Medication Works: Depresses the central nervous system to reduce anxiety or control panic.

Dosage Form and Strength:
- tablets (0.25 mg, 0.5 mg, 1 mg, 2 mg)
- oral solution (0.1 mg/mL, 1 mg/mL)

Storage:
- room temperature
- tightly closed

Administration:
- Usually taken 2 to 3 times daily.
- May be taken without regard to food.

Precautions:

Do not use if:
- you have had an allergic reaction to alprazolam or other drugs in the benzodiazepine family such as diazepam, lorazepam, or oxazepam.

Talk to your doctor if:
- you are taking other medications that may depress the central nervous system.
- you have asthma or other lung problems, kidney disease, or liver disease.
- you have been told that you snore.

Side Effects:

Major:
- confusion
- seizures
- hallucinations
- rash
- difficulty concentrating

Minor:
- dizziness
- drowsiness
- slurred speech
- blurred vision

Time Required for Drug to Take Effect: Effect occurs within hours of administration.

Symptoms of Overdose:
- continuing or worsening confusion or slurred speech
- severe weakness or drowsiness
- shortness of breath

Special Notes:
- Do not discontinue without first talking with your doctor.
- This medication may cause drowsiness. Avoid activities requiring mental alertness, such as operating a motor vehicle or operating dangerous machinery.
- Do not drink alcohol while taking this medication.

amantadine

Brand Names:
Symmetrel (DuPont)
Symadine (Solvay)

Generic Available: yes

Type of Drug: antiparkinsonian and antiviral

Used for: Treatment of Parkinson disease and parkinsonism, and prevention or treatment of influenza A.

How This Medication Works: Thought to stimulate the release of the neurotransmitter dopamine, to prolong the time dopamine remains in the brain, and to mimic the action of dopamine. As an antiviral drug, amantadine interferes with the ability of the influenza type A virus to infect human cells.

Dosage Form and Strength:
- capsules (100 mg)
- liquid/syrup (50 mg/5 mL)

Storage:
- room temperature
- tightly closed

Administration:
- Usually taken once daily in the morning.
- May take with or without food.

Precautions:
Do not use if:
- you have had an allergic reaction to amantadine.

Talk to your doctor if:
- you have ever had seizures, mental or emotional problems, heart disease, swollen ankles or feet, eczema-type rash, or kidney disease.
- you are taking hydrochlorothiazide, triamterene, antihistamines, antispasmodics (medicines for stomach cramps), metoclopramide, or antipsychotics (such as haloperidol and thioridazine).

Side Effects:
Major:
- seizures
- severe confusion
- fainting

Minor:
- drowsiness
- insomnia
- dizziness
- light-headedness
- dry mouth
- constipation
- rash on lower legs

Time Required for Drug to Take Effect: For
the flu, symptoms should improve in a few days. For
parkinsonism, improvement may take days or weeks.

Symptoms of Overdose:
- seizures
- severe confusion
- slurred speech
- hallucinations
- nightmares
- behavioral changes
- light-headedness with falls
- nausea and vomiting
- difficulty urinating

Special Notes:
- Amantadine may lose its effectiveness after
  several months.
- Patients with confusion or memory problems can
  be more sensitive to side effects of amantadine,
  which cause mental changes.
- Some patients with heart failure have experienced
  increased shortness of breath and a worsening of
  heart-failure symptoms.
- A harmless rash often occurs on the lower legs of
  people who take this medicine for a long time. It
  will disappear when the medicine is stopped.

amiodarone

Brand Name: Cordarone (Wyeth-Ayerst)

Generic Available: no

Type of Drug: antiarrhythmic

Used for: Treatment of seriously abnormal heart rhythms (atrial fibrillation, ventricular tachycardia).

How This Medication Works: Prolongs the time that the heart is in a resting phase and decreases the excitability of cardiac muscle.

Dosage Form and Strength: tablets (200 mg)

Storage:
- room temperature
- tightly closed
- protected from humidity

Administration:
- Usually prescribed once or twice daily.
- You may have to take several tablets daily for the first few weeks. This is called a loading dose.
- May be taken with food if stomach upset occurs.

Precautions:
Do not use if:
- you are allergic to amiodarone.
- medicine is beyond the expiration date.

Talk to your doctor if:
- you are taking warfarin, digoxin, phenytoin, pro-cainamide, quinidine, theophylline, or any medicine in the beta blocker family (such as atenolol, metoprolol, and propranolol).
- you have ever had heart block or a very slow heart beat.
- you have liver disease.

Side Effects:

Major:
- chest pain
- difficulty breathing
- wheezing, cough, and shortness of breath

Minor:
- dry eyes
- fatigue
- nausea
- vomiting
- constipation
- loss of appetite
- lack of coordination
- dizziness
- insomnia
- headache

Time Required for Drug to Take Effect: Starts
working in 2 to 3 days, but full effect takes 2 to 3 weeks.

Symptoms of Overdose:
- extremely slow heart beat
- low blood pressure (light-headedness, dizziness)

Special Notes:
- Your doctor will want to monitor your thyroid function while you are taking amiodarone.
- Use a sunblock with at least SPF 15 when outside because amiodarone may increase your sensitivity to the sun.
- A blue-gray discoloration of the skin may develop after prolonged treatment. This is only of cosmetic concern.

amitriptyline

Brand Names:
Elavil (Stuart)   Enovil (Hauck)
Endep (Roche)

Generic Available: yes

Type of Drug: tricyclic antidepressant

Used for: Treatment of depression and chronic pain.

How This Medication Works: Increases the
action of the neurotransmitters norepinephrine and
serotonin in the brain.

Dosage Form and Strength: tablets (10 mg,
25 mg, 50 mg, 75 mg, 100 mg, 150 mg)

Storage:
- room temperature
- tightly closed

Administration:
- Usually taken at bedtime.
- May be prescribed 2 to 3 times daily, depending
  on the dose and your response to the medicine.
- May be taken with or without food.

Precautions:
Do not use if:
- you are allergic to amitriptyline or any other tricyclic antidepressant such as imipramine.
- you are also taking an antidepressant of the
  monoamine oxidase (MAO) inhibitor type such as
  phenelzine or selegiline.

Talk to your doctor if:
- you have glaucoma (angle closure type), heart disease, urinary or prostate problems, severe constipation, breathing problems, seizures, diabetes, or a thyroid problem.
- you are taking cimetidine, clonidine, methyldopa, reserpine, guanethidine, sedatives, muscle relaxants, antihistamines, decongestants (including cold medications), stimulants.
- you drink alcohol.

Side Effects:
Major:
- dizziness with falls
- fainting
- rapid heart beat
- chest pain
- confusion
- severe constipation
- urinary retention
- rash
- severe sedation
- fever
- hallucinations
- restlessness and agitation
- severe sunburn

Minor:
- drowsiness
- dry mouth
- mild constipation
- weight gain
- unpleasant taste
- stomach upset

Time Required for Drug to Take Effect: May take from 4 to 8 weeks for full antidepressant benefit; certain types of pain may improve in 1 to 2 weeks.

Symptoms of Overdose:

- confusion
- hallucinations
- seizures
- extreme sedation
- very slow or rapid heart beat
- difficulty breathing
- inability to urinate
- severe constipation
- dilated pupils

Special Notes:

- Know which "target symptoms" (restlessness, worry, fear, or changes in sleep or appetite) you are being treated for and be prepared to tell your doctor if your target symptoms are improving, worsening, or unchanged.
- Amitriptyline can be measured in the blood. Your doctor may order a blood test to determine the level of amitriptyline in your body.
- Check with your physician or pharmacist before using any over-the-counter medications.
- Do not discontinue or increase your dose without first talking with your doctor.
- If you have diabetes you may need to check your blood glucose more frequently.
- Use a sunblock with at least SPF 15 when outside because amitriptyline may increase your sensitivity to the sun.

amlodipine

Brand Name: Norvasc (Pfizer)

Generic Available: no

Type of Drug: calcium channel blocker

Used for: Relief of angina. Sustained-release or long-acting products for treatment of high blood pressure (hypertension).

How This Medication Works: Inhibits smooth muscle contraction and causes blood vessels to dilate.

Dosage Form and Strength: tablets (2.5 mg, 5 mg, 10 mg)

Storage:
- room temperature
- protected from humidity

Administration:
- For high blood pressure, usual dosage is 5 mg once daily.
- Take at the same time every day.
- Take with food or water if stomach upset occurs.

Precautions:

Do not use if:
- you have ever had an allergic reaction to amlodipine or another calcium channel blocker such as felodipine.

Talk to your doctor if:
- you have heart disease, kidney or liver disease, or problems with circulation or your blood vessels.

- you are taking any other medications, especially medications for the heart or blood pressure such as carbamazepine, cyclosporin, or warfarin.

Side Effects:

Major:
- bleeding or bruising, especially in the gum area
- skin rash, itching
- difficulty breathing
- chest pressure or discomfort
- fainting
- swelling of ankles, feet, or lower legs

Minor:
- low blood pressure (light-headedness, dizziness)
- headache
- sexual dysfunction (impotence)
- flushing
- drowsiness
- nausea
- constipation
- tiredness

Time Required for Drug to Take Effect:

Amlodipine starts to work within 30 to 50 minutes, but it takes at least 2 to 4 weeks to see the maximal response.

Symptoms of Overdose:

- nausea
- vomiting
- weakness
- dizziness
- drowsiness

- confusion
- slurred speech
- palpitations
- loss of consciousness

Special Notes:
- Amlodipine is not a cure and you may have to take this medication for a long time.
- Changing positions slowly when sitting and/or standing up may help decrease dizziness caused by this medication.
- If you notice dizziness, avoid performing activities requiring mental alertness, such as driving a car or operating machinery.
- Constipation, a minor side effect, may be relieved by drinking more water, eating foods which are high in fiber (vegetables, fruits, bran), and exercising.
- Check with your physician or pharmacist before using any over-the-counter medications.
- Avoid becoming dehydrated or overheated. Avoid saunas, strenuous exercise in hot weather, and alcoholic beverages. Drink plenty of fluids.

amoxicillin

Brand Names:
Amoxil (SK Beecham)   Trimox (Apothecon)
Polymox (Apothecon)   Wymox (Wyeth-Ayerst)

Generic Available: yes

Type of Drug: antibiotic

Used For: Treatment of bacterial and fungal infections of the ear, respiratory tract, skin, and genitourinary tract.

How this Medication Works: Inhibits cell wall synthesis in infecting bacteria.

Dosage Form and Strength:
- tablets (125 mg, 250 mg)
- capsules (250 mg, 500 mg)
- suspension (125 mg/5 mL, 250 mg/5 mL)

Storage:
Capsules and tablets:
- room temperature
- tightly closed
- protected from humidity

Suspension:
- refrigerated
- tightly closed

Administration:
- Usually taken 3 times daily.
- May be taken without regard to meals.
- Take at even intervals, every 8 hours.
- Take until completely gone, even if symptoms have improved.
- For liquid forms, shake bottle well before measuring dose.
- Tablets may be chewed thoroughly and swallowed.

Precautions:
Do not use if:
- you are allergic to amoxicillin or penicillin.
- medicine is beyond the expiration date.

Talk to your doctor if:
- you have an allergy to cephalosporins such as cephalexin, cefaclor, cefadroxil, or cefuroxime.
- you are taking allopurinol, atenolol, or other antibiotics.

Side Effects:
Major:
- skin rash or hives
- severe diarrhea
- shortness of breath
- wheezing
- black tongue
- unusual bleeding or bruising

Minor:
- diarrhea
- abnormal taste sensation
- dry mouth
- nausea

Time Required for Drug to Take Effect:
Begins to kill bacteria within hours after your first dose. However, you must continue to take amoxicillin for the full course of treatment, even if symptoms disappear.

Symptoms of Overdose:
- hallucinations
- seizures
- lethargy
- coma

Special Notes:
- Do not use for infections other than the one for which it was prescribed.

- Discard liquid after 7 days (14 days, if refrigerated).
- Long-term treatment may lead to bacteria and fungus not sensitive to amoxicillin.

amoxicillin and clavulanic acid combination

Brand Name: Augmentin (SK Beecham)

Generic Available: no

Type of Drug: antibiotic

Used for: Treatment of bacterial and fungal infections of the ear, respiratory tract, skin, and genitourinary tract.

How This Medication Works: Inhibits cell wall synthesis in infecting bacteria. Clavulanic acid inhibits an enzyme produced by the bacteria, so antibiotic remains in the system longer.

Dosage Form and Strength:
- tablets (250 mg, 500 mg)
- suspension (125 mg/5 mL, 250 mg/5 mL)

Storage:
Capsules:
- room temperature
- tightly closed
- protected from humidity

Suspension:
- refrigerated
- tightly closed

Administration:
- Usually taken 3 times daily.
- May be taken without regard to meals.
- Take at even intervals, every 8 hours.
- Take until completely gone, even if symptoms have improved.
- Take with food if stomach upset occurs.
- For liquid, shake bottle well before measuring.

Precautions:
Do not use if:
- you are allergic to amoxicillin, clavulanic acid, or penicillin.
- medicine is beyond the expiration date.

Talk to your doctor if:
- you have an allergy to cephalosporins such as cephalexin, cefaclor, cefadroxil, or cefuroxime.
- you are taking allopurinol, atenolol, or other antibiotics.

Side Effects:
Major:
- skin rash or hives
- severe diarrhea
- shortness of breath
- wheezing
- black tongue
- unusual bleeding or bruising

Minor:
- diarrhea
- abnormal taste sensation
- dry mouth
- nausea

Time Required for Drug to Take Effect:
Begins to kill bacteria within hours after first dose. However, you must continue to take the medicine for the full course of treatment, even if symptoms disappear.

Symptoms of Overdose:
- hallucinations
- seizures
- lethargy
- coma

Special Notes:
- Do not use for infections other than the one for which it was prescribed.
- Discard any liquid medication after 10 days.
- Long-term treatment may lead to bacteria and fungus not sensitive to amoxicillin.

ampicillin

Brand Names:
Polycillin (Apothecon)   Omnipen (Wyeth-Ayerst)
Principen (Apothecon)   Totacillin (SK Beecham)

Generic Available: yes

Type of Drug: antibiotic

Used for: Treatment of bacterial and fungal infections of the ear, respiratory tract, skin, and genitourinary tract.

How This Medication Works: Inhibits cell wall synthesis in infecting bacteria.

Dosage Form and Strength:
- capsules (250 mg, 500 mg)
- suspension (250 mg/5 mL, 500 mg/5 mL)

Storage:
Capsules:
- room temperature
- tightly closed
- protected from humidity

Suspension:
- refrigerated
- tightly closed

Administration:
- Usually taken 3 to 4 times daily.
- Take on an empty stomach, 1 hour before or 2 hours after meals.
- Take at even intervals, every 6 or 8 hours, depending on number of doses.
- Take until completely gone, even if symptoms have improved.
- For liquid forms, shake bottle well before measuring dose.

Precautions:
Do not use if:
- you are allergic to ampicillin or penicillin.
- medicine is beyond the expiration date.

Talk to your doctor if:
- you have an allergy to cephalosporins such as cephalexin, cefaclor, cefadroxil, or cefuroxime.
- you are taking allopurinol, atenolol, or other antibiotics.

Side Effects:
Major:
- skin rash or hives
- severe diarrhea
- shortness of breath
- wheezing
- black tongue
- unusual bleeding or bruising

Minor:
- diarrhea
- abnormal taste sensation
- dry mouth
- nausea

Time Required for Drug to Take Effect:
Begins to kill infecting bacteria within hours after taking your first dose. However, you must continue to take ampicillin for the full course of treatment, even if symptoms disappear.

Symptoms of Overdose:
- hallucinations
- seizures
- lethargy
- coma

Special Notes:
- Do not use for infections other than the one for which it was prescribed.
- Discard liquid after 7 days (14 days, if refrigerated).
- Long-term treatment may lead to bacteria and fungus not sensitive to ampicillin.

atenolol

Brand Name: Tenormin (ICI Pharma)

Generic Available: yes

Type of Drug: beta-adrenergic blocking agent (beta blocker)

Used for: Relief of angina (chest pressure or discomfort) and treatment of high blood pressure (hypertension) and heart attacks.

How This Medication Works: Inhibits certain hormones that increase heart rate and blood pressure.

Dosage Form and Strength: tablets (25 mg, 50 mg, 100 mg)

Storage:
- room temperature
- protected from humidity

Administration:
- For high blood pressure and angina, usually taken once daily.
- Take at the same time every day.
- Administration in cases of heart attacks limited to hospital use.

Precautions:

Do not use if:
- you have ever had an allergic reaction to atenolol or another beta blocker such as metoprolol or propranolol.

Talk to your doctor if:
- you are taking any other medications.

Side Effects:

Major:
- skin rash, itching
- sexual dysfunction
- difficulty breathing
- cold hands and feet
- confusion, hallucinations, or nightmares
- palpitations or irregular heart beat
- depression or sad mood
- swelling of feet, ankles, or lower legs
- chest pressure or discomfort
- unusual bleeding or bruising

Minor:
- trouble sleeping
- low blood pressure (light-headedness, dizziness)
- drowsiness
- nervousness, anxiety
- nausea
- diarrhea
- constipation

Time Required for Drug to Take Effect: Starts
to work within 1 to 2 hours, but it takes at least 2 to
4 weeks to see the maximal response.

Symptoms of Overdose:
- slow, fast, or irregular heart beat
- fainting or severe dizziness
- difficulty breathing
- seizures or convulsions
- blue tint to nail beds or palms

Special Notes:
- Do not discontinue without your doctor's consent.
- Changing positions slowly when sitting and/or standing up may help decrease dizziness.
- If you notice dizziness, avoid activities that require mental alertness such as operating a motor vehicle or operating machinery.
- Atenolol is not a cure and you may have to take this medication for a long time.
- Check with your physician or pharmacist before using any over-the-counter medications.
- Older patients may also be more sensitive to cold temperatures while on this medication.

azithromycin

Brand Name: Zithromax (Pfizer)

Generic Available: no

Type of Drug: antibiotic

Used for: Treatment of infections of the ear, respiratory tract, skin, and genitourinary tract.

How This Medication Works: Inhibits protein synthesis in invading bacteria.

Dosage Form and Strength: capsules (250 mg)

Storage:
- room temperature
- tightly closed
- protected from humidity

Administration:
- Take 2 capsules on the first day and 1 capsule every day thereafter for 4 more days.
- Take on an empty stomach, 1 hour before or 2 hours after a meal.
- Take at the same time every day.
- Take until completely gone, even if symptoms have improved.

Precautions:
Do not use if:
- you are allergic to azithromycin or other drugs in the erythromycin family such as clarithromycin.
- medicine is beyond the expiration date.

Talk to your doctor if:
- If you are taking theophylline or warfarin.

Side Effects:
Major:
- rash
- swelling of tongue or lips
- chest pain

Minor:
- diarrhea
- nausea or abdominal pain

Time Required for Drug to Take Effect:
Begins to kill bacteria within hours after first dose. However, you must continue to take azithromycin for the full course of treatment, even if symptoms disappear.

Symptoms of Overdose:
- persistent nausea and vomiting
- severe diarrhea

Special Notes:
- Do not use for infections other than the one for which it was prescribed.
- Continues to work for several days after you finish taking it. Give azithromycin 10 days to work.
- If using antacids, separate doses of azithromycin and antacid by 2 hours.

baclofen

Brand Name: Lioresal (Ciba-Geigy)

Generic Available: yes

Type of Drug: muscle relaxant

Used for: Treatment of muscle spasticity due to multiple sclerosis, spinal cord injury, trigeminal neuralgia (tic douloureux), and tardive dyskinesia.

How This Medication Works: Interferes with the transmission of messages from the spinal cord to muscles.

Dosage Form and Strength: tablets (10 mg, 20 mg)

Storage:
- room temperature
- tightly closed

Administration:
- Initially 5 mg 2 or 3 times daily. Dose is increased gradually.

Precautions:

Do not use if:

- you have ever had an allergic reaction to baclofen.

Talk to your doctor if:

- you have ever had a stroke, brain injury, seizures.
- you are taking medicine for depression, sleep problems, allergies, or anxiety or other mental problems.
- you are taking a narcotic pain medicine such as codiene, hydrocodone, or morphine.
- you have diabetes.

Side Effects:

Major:

- seizures
- dizziness or fainting
- slurred speech
- confusion
- mental problems
- rash
- vomiting

Minor:

- drowsiness
- mild dizziness, light-headedness
- fatigue or unusual weakness
- headache
- upset stomach
- constipation
- increased urination

Time Required for Drug to Take Effect: May take days to weeks for muscle relaxation benefit.

Symptoms of Overdose:
- seizures
- coma
- extreme sedation
- decreased breathing rate
- extreme muscle weakness or twitching
- blurred vision or double vision
- vomiting

Special Notes:
- Many other medicines have similar side effects. To avoid the possibility of having side effects add up, have your doctor and pharmacist check all medicines, including over-the-counter medicines.
- Do not drink alcohol when using this medicine.
- Do not discontinue without your doctor's consent.

beclomethasone dipropionate (inhaler)

Brand Names:
Beclovent (Allen & Hansbury)
Vanceril (Schering)

Generic Available: no

Type of Drug: anti-inflammatory steroid

Used for: Treatment of asthma.

How This Medication Works: Prevents the inflammation that occurs when an allergen irritates the lungs.

Dosage Form and Strength: Inhaler
(42 μg/inhalation)

Storage:
- room temperature
- protected from humidity

Administration:
- Usually prescribed as 2 inhalations, 3 or 4 times daily.
- Allow at least 2 minutes between inhalations.
- If you have more than one inhaler, it is important to administer your inhalers in the correct order. If you are using beclomethasone and another inhaler, use the other inhaler first. Wait at least 5 minutes before inhaling beclomethasone after you have used the first medication. If you are using three classes of inhalers, use the bronchodilator (albuterol, metaproterenol), then ipratropium, and then the beclomethasone inhaler.
- Have your doctor or pharmacist demonstrate the proper procedure for using it and make sure they have you practice your technique in front of them.

Precautions:
Do not use if:
- you have an allergy to beclomethasone or other steroids such as triamcinolone, prednisone, dexamethasone, or flunisolide.

Talk to your doctor if:
- you have lung disease, bone disease, osteoporosis, diabetes, problems with your digestive

tract (ulcers, colitis, diverticulitis), infection (especially of the throat, mouth, or lungs), glaucoma or other eye disease, heart disease or high blood pressure, high blood cholesterol levels, kidney or liver disease, myasthenia gravis, or thyroid disease.
- you have had a heart attack recently.
- you are taking any other medications, especially medication for diabetes.

Side Effects:
Major:
- skin rash, hives, or itching
- difficulty breathing
- symptoms of infection
- creamy white patches inside the mouth
- irregular heartbeat
- nausea or vomiting
- decreased or blurred vision
- difficulty swallowing
- increased blood pressure
- increased thirst (severe)
- depression or mood changes
- swelling of face, feet, or lower legs
- unusual weight gain
- bloody or black, tarry stools
- back or rib pain

Minor:
- acne or other skin problems
- fullness or rounding out of the face
- menstrual problems
- muscle weakness, cramps, or pain
- upset stomach or heartburn
- bloated feeling or gas

- diarrhea or constipation
- cough
- dizziness or light-headedness
- headache
- hoarseness
- loss of appetite
- loss of smell or taste
- nervousness
- unpleasant taste
- dry, irritated mouth, tongue, or throat
- general discomfort, illness, shakiness
- increased appetite
- increased sweating
- trouble sleeping

Time Required for Drug to Take Effect: Starts
to work within minutes. However, it takes anywhere
from 1 to 4 weeks to prevent an asthma attack.

Symptoms of Overdose:
- difficulty breathing
- irregular heartbeat
- nausea or vomiting
- decreased or blurred vision
- difficulty swallowing
- increased thirst (severe)
- depression or mood changes
- swelling of face, feet, or lower legs

Special Notes:
- Sometimes a spacer device is used with your
  inhaler. This device helps the medication get to
  the lungs instead of only the mouth or throat.

- Check first with your physician and pharmacist before using any over-the-counter medications.
- Keep track of how many inhalations are left and get your medication refilled about 1 week before you expect to run out.
- Clean your inhaler every day.
- Gargle and rinse your mouth out after each use to prevent hoarseness, throat irritation, and infections in the mouth.
- Do not swallow the solution you use to rinse with because it may contain some left-over medication.
- Tell the doctor or dentist that you are taking this medication before you have any kind of surgery or emergency treatment. It may be helpful to wear an ID bracelet saying that you have asthma and are taking this type of medication.
- This medication is used to prevent an asthma attack and, therefore, it must be taken continuously. It is not effective to relieve symptoms of an acute attack, but may be used with a medication that is effective for an acute attack.

benztropine

Brand Name: Cogentin (Merck)

Generic Available: yes

Type of Drug: antiparkinsonian (anticholinergic)

Used for: Treatment of Parkinson disease and parkinsonism.

How This Medication Works: Blocks the action of the neurotransmitter acetylcholine restoring the balance between it and another neurotransmitter dopamine.

Dosage Form and Strength: tablets (0.5 mg, 1 mg, 2 mg)

Storage:
- room temperature
- tightly closed

Administration:
- Usually taken once or twice daily.
- May take with food to avoid upset stomach.

Precautions:
Do not use if:
- you have ever had an allergic reaction to benztropine.
- you have narrow-angle glaucoma (angle-closure type), colitis, severe constipation, prostate problems, myasthenia gravis, or tardive dyskinesia.

Talk to your doctor if:
- you are taking medicines for anxiety, depression, sleep problems, hallucinations, other mental conditions, dizziness, seasickness, upset stomach, cramping (muscle relaxants), hiatal hernia, allergies, irregular heart beat, or pain.
- you have dry mouth, constipation, urinary retention, breathing problems, liver disease, kidney disease, or rapid heart beat.
- you are taking metoclopramide or antipsychotics such as haloperidol and thioridazine.

Side Effects:
Major:
- eye pain
- dilated pupils
- severe constipation
- difficulty urinating
- pain when urinating
- seizures
- severe agitation
- severe confusion
- hot, dry, flushed skin
- fever
- numbness in fingers
- severe muscle weakness or cramping

Minor:
- dizziness
- drowsiness
- sedation
- dry mouth
- blurred vision
- mild constipation

Time Required for Drug to Take Effect: Relief
of symptoms occurs within 1 to 2 hours.

Symptoms of Overdose:
- eye pain
- dilated pupils
- severe constipation
- inability to urinate
- seizures
- severe confusion, agitation, or psychosis
- hyperactivity, combativeness

- hot, dry, flushed skin, or fever
- severe muscle weakness or cramping
- coma, stupor

Special Notes:

- Anticholinergic drugs are usually not recommended in older adults because they may be more sensitive to side effects.
- Many other medicines have similar side effects. To avoid the possibility of having side effects add up, have your doctor and pharmacist check all medicines, including over-the-counter medicines.
- Do not drink alcohol when using this medicine.
- Avoid staying out in the hot weather for long periods of time because this medicine may increase your risk of heat stroke.
- Do not discontinue without first talking with your doctor.

betamethasone valerate

Brand Names:

Betatrex (Savage)   Valisone (Schering)
Beta-Val (Lemmon)

Generic Available: yes

Type of Drug: topical

Used for: Treatment of dermatitis, eczema, psoriasis, poison ivy, and other skin disorders.

How This Medication Works: Relieves skin inflammation, redness, swelling, and discomfort.

Dosage Form and Strength:
- cream (0.1%, 0.01%)
- ointment (0.1%)
- lotion (0.1%)

Storage:
- room temperature
- tightly closed
- protected from humidity

Administration:
- Clean affected area with soap and water and pat dry with a clean towel (skin should be slightly moist) before application.
- Apply a thin layer to affected area twice daily or as directed.
- Do not bandage or cover unless directed by your doctor.
- Do not apply on cuts or open wounds.
- If you miss a dose of betamethasone valerate, apply the dose as soon as you remember unless it is near the time of the next dose, in which case skip the dose and return to the usual schedule.
- If using the lotion, shake the bottle well before each application.

Precautions:
Do not use if:
- you have had a severe allergic reaction to betamethasone valerate, betamethasone dipropionate, amcinonide, clocortolone, cortisone, desonide, desoximetasone, dexamethasone, diflorasone, flumethasone, fluocinolone, fluo-

cinonide, fluorometholone, flurandrenolide, halcinonide, hydrocortisone, methylprednisolone,
prednisolone, prednisone, triamcinolone, or other
steroids.

Talk to your doctor if:
- you have blood vessel disease, cataracts, diabetes, a fungal infection, glaucoma, shingles,
stomach ulcers, skin infections, or tuberculosis.

Side Effects:
Major:
- blistering
- bruising easily
- increased hair growth
- infection
- irritation
- loss of skin color or thinning of the skin

Minor:
- acne
- burning or stinging sensation
- dry or itchy skin
- redness

Time Required for Drug to Take Effect:
Symptoms usually begin to improve after 1 week.

Symptoms of Overdose: Usually not a problem
when used on the skin. If accidentally taken by mouth,
contact your doctor or a poison center for instructions.

Special Notes:
- Do not use for skin problems other than the one
for which it was prescribed.
- Do not use around the eyes.

- Keep the affected area clean and dry, wear freshly laundered clothing, and avoid tight-fitting clothing.

betaxolol

Brand Names:
Betoptic (Alcon)
Betoptic S (Alcon)

Generic Available: no

Type of Drug: topical ophthalmic agent

Used for: Treatment of glaucoma.

How This Medication Works: Lowers the fluid pressure in the eye, probably by decreasing fluid production.

Dosage Form and Strength:
- ophthalmic solution (0.25%)
- ophthalmic suspension (0.5%)

Storage:
- room temperature
- tightly closed
- protected from humidity

Administration:
- Usually prescribed as 1 or 2 drops in each eye twice daily.
- Wash your hands thoroughly with soap and water before using.

- Avoid touching the dropper tip of bottle against your eye or anything else.
- While tilting your head back, pull down the lower eyelid with your index finger to form a pocket.
- With the other hand, hold the bottle (tip down) as close to the eye as possible without touching it.
- Bracing the remaining fingers of that hand against your face, gently squeeze the dropper so that one drop falls into the pocket made by the lower eyelid.
- Close your eye gently and avoid blinking.
- The eye can hold only one drop at a time; wait at least 5 minutes between each drop.
- Replace and tighten the cap right away and do not wipe or rinse the dropper tip.
- Wash your hands to remove any medication.
- For suspensions, shake well before using.

Precautions:

Do not use if:

- you have had an allergic reaction to betaxolol or another beta blocker, such as acebutolol, atenolol, carteolol, labetalol, metoprolol, nadolol, oxprenolol, penbutolol, pindolol, propranolol, sotalol, or timolol.
- you have overt heart failure, heart block, cardiac shock, or a slow heart rate.

Talk to your doctor if:

- you have a history of heart block or heart failure.
- you have diabetes, overactive thyroid (hyperthyroidism), myasthenia gravis, breathing problems, peripheral vascular disease, or poor circulation.

- you are taking any other medication, especially reserpine or beta blockers such as acebutolol, atenolol, carteolol, labetalol, metoprolol, nadolol, oxprenolol, penbutolol, pindolol, pro-pranolol, sotalol, or timolol.

Side Effects:
Major:
- severe irritation or inflammation of eye or eyelid
- confusion
- depression
- slow heart beat
- trouble sleeping
- unusual tiredness or weakness
- wheezing or trouble breathing
- dizziness
- headache
- hives
- redness or irritation of the tongue

Minor:
- stinging of the eye or other irritation during administration

Time Required for Drug to Take Effect:
Begins to work immediately; however, glaucoma returns to pretreatment levels when medication is stopped.

Symptoms of Overdose:
- heart failure
- slow heart rate
- heart block
- wheezing or trouble breathing

Special Notes:
- Eye drops are hard to use; have someone help you if possible. Tell your doctor if you cannot put them in yourself and have no one to help you.
- Tell the doctor or dentist that you are taking this medication before any kind of treatment.
- May cause light sensitivity; use sunglasses.
- If betaxolol is replacing another eye drop, continue the other drop during the first day of betaxolol treatment and stop the second day.

bethanechol

Brand Names:
Urecholine (Merck)
Duvoid (Roberts)

Generic Available: yes

Type of Drug: Cholinergic stimulant

Used for: Treatment of urine retention or incontinence.

How This Medication Works: Improves the muscle tone of the urinary bladder.

Dosage Form and Strength: tablets (10 mg, 25 mg, 50 mg)

Storage:
- room temperature
- tightly closed
- protected from humidity

Administration:
- Doses may vary; usual dose is 25 to 50 mg 3 or 4 times daily, starting with 5 to 10 mg every 6 hours until the desired response or 50-mg dose is reached.
- If you forget a dose, take it as soon as you remember if it is less than 2 hours after the dose was scheduled. If it is 2 or more hours after the dose was scheduled, skip the missed dose and take the next dose at the regular time.

Precautions:
Do not use if:
- you have had a previous allergic reaction to bethanechol.
- you have anastomosis.
- you have had recent bladder or stomach surgery.

Talk to your doctor if:
- you regularly experience light-headedness, dizziness, or fainting on standing.
- you have asthma, slow heart rate, low blood pressure, angina, overactive thyroid, stomach ulcers.
- you are taking any medication, especially quinidine and procainamide.

Side Effects:
Major:
- wheezing, shortness of breath, or chest tightness
- seizures

Minor:
- belching
- blurred vision
- diarrhea
- dizziness, light-headedness, or fainting

- frequent urge to urinate
- headache
- increased saliva
- increased sweating
- sleeplessness or nervousness
- stomach pain

Time Required for Drug to Take Effect: Effects appear within 30 to 90 minutes after dose.

Symptoms of Overdose:
- cardiac collapse
- bloody diarrhea
- low blood pressure (dizziness, light-headedness)
- cardiac arrest

Special Notes:
- Taking bethanechol on an empty stomach (1 hour before meals) reduces the chance of an upset stomach or vomiting.
- Do not discontinue without talking to your doctor.

bromocriptine

Brand Name: Parlodel (Sandoz)

Generic Available: no

Type of Drug: antiparkinsonian

Used for: Treatment of Parkinson disease.

How This Medication Works: Mimics the action of the neurotransmitter dopamine, which is lacking in Parkinson disease.

Dosage Form and Strength:
- tablets (2.5 mg)
- capsules (5 mg)

Storage:
- room temperature
- tightly closed

Administration:
- Initially taken 1 or 2 times daily.
- May increase to 3 times daily after several weeks.
- Take with meals to prevent stomach upset.

Precautions:
Do not use if:
- you have ever had an allergic reaction to bromocriptine or other ergot alkaloids.

Talk to your doctor if:
- you have heart disease, high blood pressure (hypertension), or circulation problems.
- you experience confusion or memory problems.
- you are taking metoclopramide or antipsychotics such as haloperidol or thioridazine.

Side Effects:
Major:
- seizures
- severe nausea and vomiting
- chest pain
- fainting
- severe agitation or confusion
- difficulty breathing
- vision changes
- black, tarry stools

Minor:
- stomach upset
- dizziness
- light-headedness when sitting up or standing up
- cold sensitivity in fingers and toes
- hallucinations
- constipation or diarrhea
- dry mouth
- stuffy nose

Time Required for Drug to Take Effect: Takes weeks to months for maximum benefit because bromocriptine doses must be increased very slowly.

Symptoms of Overdose:
- seizures
- fainting
- severe nausea
- extreme agitation
- hallucinations

Special Notes:
- When bromocriptine is added to your regimen, the doctor may adjust the doses of your other medications as you begin to respond. If you are having difficulty keeping track of your medication schedule, talk with your doctor or pharmacist. Skipping doses or accidentally taking extra doses can be dangerous.
- Patients who have some confusion, emotional problems, or memory problems may be more sensitive to this medicine. If you notice any changes in behavior or emotions, talk with your doctor.

bumetanide

Brand Name: Bumex (Roche)

Generic Available: no

Type of Drug: diuretic

Used for: Treatment of edema (fluid retention) and high blood pressure (hypertension).

How This Medication Works: Inhibits sodium reabsorption in a specific part of the kidney, resulting in loss of water through urine.

Dosage Form and Strength: tablets (0.5 mg, 1 mg, 2 mg)

Storage:
- room temperature
- tightly closed
- protected from humidity

Administration:
- Usually taken once daily, in the morning.
- Take with food or milk if stomach upset occurs.

Precautions:
Do not use if:
- you are allergic to bumetanide or to oral diabetes medication such as glipizide or glyburide.

Talk to your doctor if:
- you have liver disease, coronary artery disease, or gout.
- you are taking digoxin, an angiotensin-converting enzyme (ACE) inhibitor (such as captopril, enalapril,

or lisinopril) a thiazide diuretic (such as hydrochlorothiazide, chlorthalidone, or metolazone),
warfarin, lithium, theophylline, propranolol,
chloral hydrate, phenytoin, aspirin, a nonsteroidal
anti-inflammatory drug (such as ibuprofen, piroxicam, diclofenac, naproxen, or oxaprozin), or oral
diabetes medication (such as chlorpropamide,
tolazamide, glipizide, or glyburide).
• you have had a heart attack.

Side Effects:
Major:
  • profound dehydration (thirst, rapid heart beat,
    weakness, fatigue, drowsiness, and dizziness)
  • difficulty breathing
  • muscle pain or cramps
  • fainting
  • chest pain
  • prolonged vomiting or diarrhea
  • hearing loss
Minor:
  • ringing in the ears (tinnitus)
  • dizziness
  • dry mouth
  • upset stomach
  • headache

Time Required for Drug to Take Effect:
Begins to work in 30 to 60 minutes and its effects last
about 6 hours.

Symptoms of Overdose:
  • acute and profound water loss
  • loss of appetite

- vomiting
- mental confusion
- weakness or lethargy
- dizziness

Special Notes:
- Take with orange juice or a banana to help replace lost potassium.
- Unless otherwise instructed by your doctor, it is important to drink 6 to 8 eight-ounce glasses of water daily to avoid dehydration.
- Use a sunblock with at least SPF 15 when outside because bumetanide may increase your sensitivity to the sun.
- If you experience dryness of the mouth, try sugar-less candy or gum, ice chips, or a saliva substitute.
- Weigh yourself daily. If you gain or lose more than 1 pound daily, call your doctor.
- Your doctor will check calcium and magnesium levels to determine if you need supplementation.
- Changing positions slowly when sitting and/or standing up may help decrease dizziness caused by this medication.
- If you have diabetes, you may need to check your blood glucose more frequently.

bupropion

Brand Name: Wellbutrin (Burroughs Wellcome)

Generic Available: no

Type of Drug: antidepressant

Used for: Treatment of depression.

How This Medication Works: Has a mild effect on several neurotransmitters in the brain.

Dosage Form and Strength: tablets (75 mg, 100 mg)

Storage:
- room temperature
- tightly closed
- protected from humidity

Administration:
- Initially taken twice daily.
- Usually increased to 3 times daily, over time.
- Usually taken in the morning, at midday, and in the evening (4 to 6 hours apart).
- May be taken with food to reduce stomach upset.

Precautions:
Do not use if:
- you are allergic to bupropion.
- you are taking a monoamine oxidase (MAO) inhibitor or if you have taken an MAO inhibitor within the past 14 days.

Talk to your doctor if:
- you have ever had seizures, taken medicine for seizures, had a serious head injury or brain tumor, had hepatitis or other liver problems, or had serious problems with your kidneys.
- you are currently taking other medicines for depression, sleep problems, or other mental conditions.

Side Effects:

Major:
- seizures
- unusual agitation or restlessness
- hallucinations
- severe confusion
- rapid heart beat
- chest pain
- difficulty breathing
- extreme drowsiness
- rash, hives, itching
- severe headache

Minor:
- drowsiness
- sleep problems
- tremor
- nausea, vomiting
- decreased appetite, weight loss
- increased appetite, weight gain
- dry mouth
- sweating
- blurred vision
- ringing in ears

Time Required for Drug to Take Effect: Full
benefit may take from 4 to 8 weeks to occur. (Should you need several dose changes, it may take even more time to get the maximum benefit of your medicine.)

Symptoms of Overdose:
- seizures
- difficulty breathing
- chest pains

- hallucinations
- loss of consciousness

Special Notes:

- Know which "target symptoms" (restlessness, worry, fear, or changes in sleep or appetite) you are being treated for and be prepared to tell your doctor if your target symptoms are improving, worsening, or if they are unchanged.
- Show your doctor and pharmacist a complete list of all medications, including over-the-counter medications that you take regularly or on occasion.
- Do not drink alcohol when using this medicine.
- Do not discontinue without first talking with your doctor.
- Never increase your dose without the advice of your doctor.

buspirone

Brand Name: BuSpar (Mead Johnson)

Generic Available: no

Type of Drug: antianxiety

Used for: Treatment of anxiety disorders and depression with anxiety

How This Medication Works: Exact mechanism is unknown, but may act by increasing levels of the neurotransmitters dopamine and norepinephrine.

Dosage Form and Strength: tablets (5 mg, 10 mg)

Storage:
- room temperature
- tightly closed
- protected from humidity

Administration:
- Usually taken 2 to 3 times daily.
- Be consistent: Either always take on an empty stomach, or always take with food.
- If you miss a dose, take it as soon as possible. Unless it is almost time for your next dose, in which case skip the missed dose.

Precautions:
Do not use if:
- you've ever had an allergic reaction to buspirone.

Talk to your doctor if:
- you have kidney or liver disease.
- you are taking a monoamine oxidase (MAO) inhibitor, haloperidol, or trazodone.

Side Effects:
Major:
- confusion
- muscle weakness
- sore throat with fever

Minor:
- dizziness or restlessness
- headache
- nausea

Time Required for Drug to Take Effect: May
take 1 to 2 weeks before any effect on anxiety is seen; optimum effects seen after 3 to 4 weeks.

Symptoms of Overdose:
- severe dizziness or drowsiness
- nausea or vomiting

Special Notes:
- Do not discontinue without first talking to your doctor.

butalbital and acetaminophen combination
butalbital, acetaminophen, and caffeine combination

Brand Names:

Without caffeine:
Bancap (Forest)
Bucet (UAD)
Phrenilin (Carnrick)
Phrenilin Forte (Carnrick)
Sedapap–10 (Mayrand)
Triaprin (Dunhall)
Tencon (Inter Ethical Labs)

With caffeine:
Fioricet (Sandoz)
Esgic (Forest)
Repan (Everett)
Amaphen (Trimen)
Butace (American Urol)
Endolor (Keene)
Medigesic (US Pharm)

Generic Available: yes

Type of Drug: analgesic

Used for: Relief of body pain and headaches.

How This Medication Works: Butalbital decreases the central nervous system's recognition of pain impulses. Acetaminophen blocks pain impulses in the peripheral nervous system. Caffeine is a central nervous system stimulant, which increases the pain-relieving effects of analgesics and decreases the amount of time before the medicine takes effect.

Dosage Form and Strength:
butalbital and acetaminophen combination:
- tablets (50 mg/325 mg, 50 mg/650 mg)
- capsules (50 mg/325 mg, 50 mg/650 mg)

butalbital, acetaminophen, and caffeine combination:
- tablets (50 mg/325 mg/40 mg)
- capsules (50 mg/325 mg/40 mg)

Storage:
- room temperature
- protected from humidity

Administration:
- Take this medication as prescribed and do not exceed the maximum number of doses per day.
- Never take more tablets per dose or more doses per day than your doctor has prescribed.
- Take with milk or food if stomach upset occurs.

Precautions:
Do not use if:
- you are allergic to butalbital, barbiturates (such as phenobarbital), caffeine, or acetaminophen.

Talk to your doctor if:
- you have anemia, depression, kidney disease, liver disease, thyroid disease, porphyria, adrenal disease, asthma, emphysema, other chronic lung conditions, or diabetes.

- you are taking naltrexone, zidovudine, or any other medications, especially those that can cause drowsiness, such as antihistamines, barbiturates (phenobarbital), benzodiazepines (diazepam, alprazolam, and lorazepam), muscle relaxants, or antidepressants.

Side Effects:

Major:
- skin rash or hives
- bleeding sores on lips
- unexplained muscle or joint pain
- abnormal heart rhythm
- sores, ulcers, or white spots in mouth
- yellow eyes or skin (jaundice)
- severe confusion
- persistent nausea or vomiting
- swelling, pain, or tenderness in the upper abdomen or stomach area
- unusual movements of the eyes

Minor:
- mild dizziness or light-headedness
- mild drowsiness
- hangover-type effect
- mild anxiety or nervousness
- constipation
- feeling faint
- headache
- nightmares

Time Required for Drug to Take Effect: Starts
to work within 40 to 60 minutes; combination with caffeine may start to work within 30 to 45 minutes.

Symptoms of Overdose:
- severe drowsiness
- unconsciousness
- shortness of breath or difficulty breathing
- unusually slow heart beat
- slurred speech
- staggering

(Symptoms associated with acetaminophen may not occur until 2 to 4 days after the overdose is taken, but it is important to begin treatment as soon as possible after the overdose to prevent liver damage or death.)

Special Notes:
- This medication may cause drowsiness. Use caution when operating a motor vehicle or operating dangerous machinery.
- Check with your physician or pharmacist before using any over-the-counter medications.
- When butalbital is used over a long period of time, your body may become tolerant and require larger doses.
- Do not stop taking this medication abruptly.
- Do not drink alcohol while taking this medication.

calcitonin

Brand Names:
Human:
Cibacalcin (Ciba-Geigy)
Salmon:
Calcimar (Rhone-Poulenc Rorer)
Miacalcin (Sandoz)

Generic Available: no

Type of Drug: hormone

Used for: Treatment of Paget disease and high blood calcium levels (hypercalcemia), and prevention of bone loss in osteoporosis.

How This Medication Works: Lowers calcium levels by preventing bone loss and increasing kidney removal of calcium.

Dosage Form and Strength:
- human: injection (500 µg/mL)
- salmon: injection (200 IU/mL)

Storage:
Human:
- room temperature below 77°F (Do not refrigerate.)
- protected from light

Salmon:
- refrigerated (Do not freeze.)
- protected from light

Administration:
Human:
- For Paget disease, usually 500 µg by subcutaneous injection daily. Sometimes 500 µg 2 or 3 times a week or 250 µg daily.

Salmon:
- For Paget disease, usually starts with 100 IU by subcutaneous or intramuscular injection and is decreased to 50 IU once daily, every other day, or 3 times a week.

- For osteoporosis, usually 100 IU by injection once a day, every other day, or 3 times a week.
- For hypercalcemia, dose is adjusted by weight and given by injection every 6 to 12 hours.

If you missed a dose:
- If you take 2 doses daily and remember within 2 hours of the missed dose, take it then and resume regular schedule. If it is 2 hours after the missed dose, skip the dose and resume the regular schedule; do not double the dose.
- If you take 1 dose daily and you remember the day the dose is missed, take it then and resume regular schedule. If it is the next day after the missed dose, skip the dose and resume the regular schedule; do not double the dose.
- If you take 1 dose every other day and remember the day the dose is missed, take it and resume regular schedule. If it is the next day, take the dose and restart the every-other-day schedule.
- If you take 1 dose 3 times a week and you miss a dose, take it the next day, set the next doses that week back a day, and resume the regular schedule the next week.

Precautions:

Do not use if:
- you have had a severe allergic or unusual reactions to calcitonin.

Talk to your doctor if:
- you have any allergies or unusual reactions to foods, preservatives, dyes, proteins, or vitamin D.
- you are taking any medications (prescription or over-the-counter).

Side Effects:

Major:
- hives, swelling, skin rash (allergic reaction)

Minor:
- loss of appetite
- diarrhea
- flushing, redness, or tingling of the face, ears, hands, or feet
- nausea or vomiting
- stomach pain
- injection-site redness, pain, or swelling
- taste changes
- increased urination frequency

Time Required for Drug to Take Effect:

Usually starts working in the first month or so of treatment but may take up to 6 months.

Special Notes:

- Once the human solution is mixed it must be used within 6 hours.
- Do not use if there are particles floating in the solution; use only when the solution is clear and colorless.

calcitriol

Brand Name: Rocaltrol (Roche)

Generic Available: yes

Type of Drug: nutritional supplement (form of vitamin D)

Used for: Treatment of bone diseases, hypoparathyroidism, and low blood calcium levels (hypocalcemia) in dialysis patients.

How This Medication Works: Keeps bones strong and keeps blood calcium levels normal.

Dosage Form and Strength: capsules (0.25 µg, 0.5 µg)

Storage:
- room temperature
- tightly closed
- protected from light

Administration:
- Usually prescribed at 0.25 µg to 3 µg daily.
- May be taken without regard to meals.
- Do not crush or chew capsules.
- If you miss a dose, take it as soon as you remember. If it is time for the next dose, take the normal dose; do not double the dose.

Precautions:
Do not use if:
- you have had a serious allergic reaction to calcitriol, calcifediol, dihydrotachysterol, or vitamin D.
- you have high blood calcium (hypercalcemia).
Talk to your doctor if:
- you have seizures or epilepsy, high blood phosphate levels (hyperphosphatemia), heart disease, renal disease, or sarcoidosis.
- you are taking any medication, especially verapamil, diuretics (such as hydrochlorothiazide),

vitamin D, dihydrotachysterol, calcifediol, cholestyramine, colestipol, mineral oil or antacids with magnesium or calcium.

Side Effects:

Major:
- decreased appetite
- bone or muscle pain
- constipation or diarrhea
- dry mouth
- eye irritation
- headache
- irregular heart beat
- itchy skin
- lethargy (unusual tiredness or weakness)
- light sensitivity
- mood changes
- nausea and vomiting
- increased thirst
- increased urination frequency
- changed urination amount
- weight loss

Minor: none

Time Required for Drug to Take Effect:
Depends on the type and severity of the problem.

Symptoms of Overdose: Same as major side effects.

Special Notes:
- Carefully follow any special diet or calcium sup-plementation recommendations your doctor has given you.

captopril

Brand Name: Capoten (Bristol-Myers Squibb)

Generic Available: yes

Type of Drug: antihypertensive (angiotensin-converting enzyme [ACE] inhibitor)

Used for: Treatment of high blood pressure (hypertension), congestive heart failure, and kidney disease caused by diabetes (diabetic nephropathy), and preservation of heart function after a heart attack.

How This Medication Works: Inhibits enzyme necessary for the formation of angiotensin, a substance that causes powerful constriction of blood vessels.

Dosage Form and Strength: tablets (12.5 mg, 25 mg, 50 mg, 100 mg)

Storage:
- room temperature
- tightly closed
- protected from humidity

Administration:
- Usually taken 2 to 3 times daily.
- Best taken on an empty stomach.
- Take at least 1 hour before or 2 hours after taking antacids.

Precautions:
Do not use if:
- you are allergic to captopril or other ACE inhibitors such as enalapril or lisinopril.

- you have liver disease (bilateral renal artery stenosis).

Talk to your doctor if:
- you are taking a diuretic (such as hydrochloro-thiazide or furosemide), a potassium supplement indomethacin, any nonsteroidal anti-inflamma-tory drug (such as aspirin, ibuprofen, naproxen, piroxicam, or ketoprofen), allopurinol, digoxin, lithium, or probenecid.
- you have kidney disease.

Side Effects:
Major:
- swelling of the mouth, lips, or tongue
- fainting
- generalized rash
- chest pain
- irregular heart beat

Minor:
- cough
- taste disturbances
- headache
- dizziness or fatigue
- impotence or decreased sexual desire

Time Required for Drug to Take Effect:
Usually starts to work after about 1 week of therapy, but sometimes several weeks of therapy are needed for it to reach its maximum effect.

Symptoms of Overdose:
- very low blood pressure
- profound muscle weakness
- nausea, vomiting, diarrhea

Special Notes:
- Avoid salt substitutes containing potassium.
- You will need tests to monitor kidney function and electrolytes (sodium, potassium) in the blood.
- Avoid the use of aspirin or other nonsteroidal anti-inflammatory drugs such as ibuprofen or naproxen. Use acetaminophen for pain relief.
- May cause a dry cough. Talk to your doctor if you develop a particularly bothersome cough.
- Use a sunblock with at least SPF 15 when outside because captopril may increase your sensitivity to the sun.

carbamazepine

Brand Names:
Tegretol (Ciba-Geigy)
Epitol (Lemmon)

Generic Available: yes

Type of Drug: anticonvulsant

Used for: Treatment of seizures, epilepsy, and trigeminal neuralgia.

How This Medication Works: Interferes with abnormal electrical activity in the brain to reduce the frequency of seizures.

Dosage Form and Strength:
- tablets (200 mg)
- chewable tablets (100 mg)
- liquid/oral suspension (100 mg/5 mL)

Storage:
Tablets:
- tightly closed
- protected from humidity

Liquid:
- room temperature
- tightly closed

Administration:
- Dose based on measurement of amount of medication in the blood.
- Take with meals.
- For liquid forms, shake well before use.
- Chewable tablets may be chewed or swallowed whole.

Precautions:
Do not use if:
- you are allergic to carbamazepine or tricyclic antidepressants (such as amitriptyline, amoxapine, or desipramine).

Talk to your doctor if:
- you have angina, coronary artery disease, liver disease, glaucoma, or severe kidney disease.
- you have ever had a heart attack, cirrhosis of the liver, or hepatitis.
- you are currently taking any other seizure medication (such as phenytoin, phenobarbital, primidone, or valproic acid), cimetidine, diltiazem, erythromycin, propoxyphene, verapamil, haloperidol, lithium, or theophylline.
- you experience symptoms of confusion or nervousness.

Side Effects:
Major:
- blurred or double vision
- skin rash
- confusion or agitation
- severe nausea
- severe drowsiness

Minor:
- mild light-headedness
- mild nausea
- constipation or diarrhea
- sensitivity of skin to sunlight

Time Required for Drug to Take Effect: Starts
acting in first few hours and decreases the number and frequency of seizures as long as it is continued.

Symptoms of Overdose:
- decrease in amount of urine
- severe nausea and vomiting
- clumsiness
- dizziness
- irregular breathing
- increased heart rate

Special Notes:
- Mild stomach upset may be minimized by taking medication with food.
- Do not stop taking this medication or change doses without first talking with your physician. More severe and frequent seizures may occur when suddenly discontinuing or altering the dosage of this medication.

- Do not use any over-the-counter medications unless you check first with your physician and pharmacist.
- Use a sunblock with at least SPF 15 when outside because carbamazepine may increase your sensitivity to the sun.

carisoprodol
carisoprodol and aspirin combination
carisoprodol, aspirin, and codeine combination

Brand Names:
Soma (Wallace)
Soma Compound (Wallace)

Soma Compound with Codeine (Wallace)

Generic Available:
- carisoprodol: yes
- carisoprodol and aspirin combination: yes
- carisoprodol, aspirin, and codeine combination: no

Type of Drug: muscle relaxant (aspirin and codeine added as analgesics)

Used for: Relief of muscle spasms due to injury.

How This Medication Works: The exact mechanism by which this medicine works is not understood, but it appears to interfere with certain neural impulses to produce relaxation of skeletal muscles.

Dosage Form and Strength:
- carisoprodol: tablets (350 mg)
- carisoprodol and aspirin combination: tablets (200 mg/325 mg)
- carisoprodol, aspirin, and codeine combination: tablets (200 mg/325 mg/16 mg)

Storage:
- room temperature
- tightly closed

Administration:
- carisoprodol: 1 tablet 3 to 4 times daily.
- carisoprodol and aspirin combination: 1 or 2 tablets 3 to 4 times daily.
- carisoprodol, aspirin, and codeine combination: 1 or 2 tablets 3 to 4 times daily.

Precautions:
Do not use if:
- you have ever had an allergic reaction to this medicine or to meprobamate.
- you have ever had an allergic reaction to aspirin or codeine (or other narcotics).
- you have porphyria.

Talk to your doctor if:
- you are taking medicines that cause drowsiness such as antihistamines; medicines for sleep, depression, or mental problems; medicines for seizures or pain; or other muscle relaxants.
- you are taking clindamycin.

Side Effects:

Major:
- severe skin rash
- difficulty breathing
- swelling around mouth and tongue
- fever
- fainting
- rapid heart beat

Minor:
- drowsiness or fatigue
- dizziness or light-headedness
- tremor
- clumsiness
- agitation or unusual behavior
- headache
- facial flushing
- vision changes
- nausea or vomiting

Time Required for Drug to Take Effect: Starts to work within 30 to 60 minutes.

Symptoms of Overdose:
- extreme drowsiness
- very low blood pressure (dizziness, fainting)
- very slow breathing

Special Notes:
- This medicine is used in addition to rest, physical therapy, or other treatment prescribed by your doctor.
- Check with your physician or pharmacist before using any other medications.

- Combination with codeine may cause constipation.
- Do not drink alcohol when using this medicine.

cefuroxime

Brand Name: Ceftin (Glaxo Wellcome)

Generic Available: no

Type of Drug: antibiotic

Used for: Treatment of infections of the ear, respiratory tract, bone, skin, and genitourinary tract.

How This Medication Works: Inhibits cell wall synthesis in infecting bacteria.

Dosage Form and Strength:
- tablets (125 mg, 250 mg, 500 mg)
- suspension (125 mg/5 mL)

Storage:
- room temperature (suspension may be refrigerated)
- tightly closed
- protected from humidity

Administration:
- Usually taken twice daily.
- Take until completely gone, even if symptoms have improved.
- Take at even intervals, every 12 hours.
- Tablets may be taken without regard to meals.
- Suspension must be taken with food.
- Shake suspension well before each use.

Precautions:

Do not use if:

- you are allergic to cefuroxime or other cephalosporins such as cephalexin, cefaclor, or cefadroxil.
- medicine is beyond the expiration date.

Talk to your doctor if:

- you are allergic to penicillin or drugs in the penicillin class such as ampicillin, and amoxicillin.
- you are taking probenecid.

Side Effects:

Major:

- skin rash or hives
- severe diarrhea
- shortness of breath or wheezing
- unusual bleeding or bruising

Minor:

- mild diarrhea
- abnormal taste sensation
- nausea
- headache

Time Required for Drug to Take Effect:

Begins to kill infecting bacteria within hours after taking your first dose. However, you must continue to take cefuroxime for the full course of treatment, even if symptoms disappear.

Symptoms of Overdose: seizures

Special Notes:

- Do not use for infections other than the one for which it was prescribed.

- Discard liquid after 10 days.
- Long-term treatment with this antibiotic may lead to the development of bacteria and fungus not sensitive to cefuroxime.

cephalexin

Brand Names:
Keflex (Dista)
Keflet (Dista)

Generic Available: yes

Type of Drug: antibiotic

Used for: Treatment of infections of the ear, respiratory tract, skin, bone, and genitourinary tract.

How This Medication Works: Inhibits cell wall synthesis in infecting bacteria.

Dosage Form and Strength:
- tablets (250 mg, 500 mg, 1 g)
- capsules (250 mg, 500 mg)
- suspension (125 mg/5 mL, 250 mg/5 mL)

Storage:
Capsules and tablets:
- room temperature
- tightly closed
- protected from humidity

Suspension:
- refrigerated
- tightly closed

Administration:
- Take at even intervals.
- May be taken without regard to meals.
- For suspension, shake well before each use.
- Take until completely gone, even if symptoms have improved.

Precautions:
Do not use if:
- you are allergic to cephalexin or other cephalosporins such as cefuroxime, cefaclor, or cefadroxil.
- medicine is beyond the expiration date.

Talk to your doctor if:
- you are allergic to penicillin or drugs in the penicillin class (such as ampicillin and amoxicillin).
- you are taking probenecid.

Side Effects:
Major:
- skin rash or hives
- severe diarrhea
- shortness of breath or wheezing
- unusual bleeding or bruising

Minor:
- diarrhea
- abnormal taste sensation
- nausea
- headache

Time Required for Drug to Take Effect:
Begins to kill infecting bacteria within hours after taking your first dose. However, you must continue to

take cephalexin for the full course of treatment, even if symptoms disappear.

Symptoms of Overdose: seizures

Special Notes:
- Do not use for infections other than the one for which it was prescribed.
- Discard liquid after 14 days.
- Long-term treatment may lead to bacteria not sensitive to cephalexin.

chloral hydrate

Brand Name: Noctec (Squibb Mark)

Generic Available: yes

Type of Drug: sedative/hypnotic

Used for: Treatment of insomnia and preoperative anxiety and prevention or suppression of alcohol withdrawal symptoms.

How This Medication Works: Exact mechanism is unknown.

Dosage Form and Strength:
- capsules (250 mg, 500 mg)
- oral syrup (250 mg/5 mL, 500 mg/5 mL)
- rectal suppositories (325 mg, 500 mg, 650 mg)

Storage:
- room temperature
- tightly closed

Administration:

- Swallow capsules whole, do not crush or chew.
- Take capsules with a full glass of water or juice.
- Dilute oral syrup in clear liquid such as water or apple juice.
- If suppository is soft, run it under cold water or refrigerate until firm.

Precautions:

Do not use if:

- you are allergic to chloral hydrate.

Talk to your doctor if:

- you are taking warfarin, phenytoin, or any medicine for depression, anxiety, insomnia, or pain.
- you have liver disease, stomach ulcers, or severe heart disease.

Side Effects:

Major:

- skin rash
- confusion
- hallucinations

Minor:

- nausea and vomiting
- diarrhea
- drowsiness
- clumsiness

Time Required for Drug to Take Effect: Starts to cause drowsiness within 30 minutes.

Symptoms of Overdose:

- confusion
- seizures

- severe drowsiness
- nausea
- vomiting
- weakness
- slurred speech

Special Notes:

- This medication causes drowsiness. Use caution when operating a motor vehicle or operating dangerous machinery.
- Do not discontinue without first talking with your doctor. Chloral hydrate can be habit forming.
- Do not drink alcohol while taking this medication.
- Side effects of nausea and vomiting will usually go away during treatment. If these continue, talk with your physician.
- Taking this medication with juice or food may lessen stomach upset.

chlordiazepoxide

Brand Names:
Libritabs (Roche)
Librium (Roche)

Generic Available: yes

Type of Drug: antianxiety

Used for: Treatment of anxiety and prevention or suppression of alcohol withdrawal symptoms.

How This Medication Works: Depresses the central nervous system.

Dosage Form and Strength:
- tablets (5 mg, 10 mg, 25 mg)
- capsules (5 mg, 10 mg, 25 mg)

Storage:
- room temperature
- tightly closed

Administration:
- Usually taken 3 to 4 times daily.
- May be taken with food or water if stomach upset occurs.
- Take chlordiazepoxide at least 1 hour before or 2 hours after taking antacids.

Precautions:
Do not use if:
- you've ever had an allergic reaction to chlordiazepoxide or drugs in the benzodiazepine family, such as diazepam, lorazepam, and oxazepam.

Talk to your doctor if:
- you are taking other medications that may depress the central nervous system, such as medicine for depression, anxiety, insomnia, or pain.
- you have asthma or other lung problems, kidney disease, or liver disease.
- you have been told that you snore.
- you are taking cimetidine, disulfiram, digoxin, fluoxetine, isoniazid, ketoconazole, levodopa, metoprolol, propoxyphene, propranolol, phenytoin, probenecid, rifampin, theophylline, or valproic acid.

Side Effects:
Major:
- seizures or hallucinations
- rash
- confusion or difficulty concentrating

Minor:
- unsteadiness or drowsiness
- slurred speech or blurred vision

Time Required for Drug to Take Effect: Starts
after first dose, but optimal effect usually occurs after
approximately 1 week of therapy.

Symptoms of Overdose:
- continuing confusion and/or slurred speech
- severe weakness or drowsiness
- shortness of breath

Special Notes:
- This medication may cause drowsiness. Use
  caution when operating a motor vehicle or operating dangerous machinery.
- Do not discontinue without first talking with your
  doctor. Chlordiazepoxide can be habit forming.
- Do not drink alcohol while taking this medication.

chlorpromazine

Brand Name: Thorazine (SK Beecham)

Generic Available: yes

Type of Drug: antipsychotic

Used for: Treatment of psychotic disorders (schizophrenia), agitation (symptoms of dementia such as hallucinations, suspiciousness, and hostility), Tourette syndrome, Huntington chorea, nausea and vomiting, and hiccups.

How This Medication Works: Blocks transmission of the neurotransmitter dopamine in the central nervous system.

Dosage Form and Strength:
- tablets (10 mg, 25 mg, 50 mg, 100 mg, 200 mg)
- extended-release capsules (30 mg, 75 mg, 150 mg, 200 mg, 300 mg)
- oral concentrate (30 mg/1 mL, 100 mg/1 mL)
- oral syrup (10 mg/5 mL)
- rectal suppositories (25 mg, 100 mg)

Storage:
Tablets, extended-release capsules, rectal suppositories:
- room temperature
- tightly closed

Oral concentrate, oral syrup:
- room temperature
- tightly closed
- protected from light

Administration:
Tablets, extended-release capsules:
- Usually taken 1 to 3 times daily.
- Swallow capsule whole, do not chew.

Oral concentrate:
- Usually taken 2 to 4 times daily

- Dilute dose in approximately 120 mL (half a tall glass) of water, juice, or other beverage before taking. Semi solid foods (gelatin, pudding, applesauce) may also be used.

Rectal suppositories:
- Usually inserted every 6 to 8 hours as needed.
- Remove foil prior to insertion.
- If suppository is soft, run it under cold water or refrigerate until firm.

Precautions:

Do not use if:
- you have had an allergic reaction to chlorpromazine or other medications from the phenothiazine family such as fluphenazine or thioridazine.
- you have Parkinson disease.

Talk to your doctor if:
- you are taking any other medication, especially lithium, guanethidine, meperidine, methyldopa, propranolol, antacids, antidiarrheals, or medication for seizures or depression.
- you have liver disease, stomach ulcers, seizures, enlarged prostate, or angina.
- you have ever had a heart attack.

Side Effects:

Major:
- blurred vision
- skin rash or sunburn
- problems speaking or swallowing
- lip smacking
- restlessness

Minor:
- constipation
- dizziness or drowsiness
- dry mouth
- urinary retention

Time Required for Drug to Take Effect: Takes several weeks before desired effect is seen.

Symptoms of Overdose:
- extreme drowsiness
- agitation or restlessness
- seizures
- fever

Special Notes:
- Oral dosage forms (tablets, capsules, liquid) may be taken with food if stomach upset occurs.
- Chlorpromazine may cause movement disorders. Tell your doctor about any involuntary muscle movements or spasms.
- Avoid contact of concentrate with skin.
- Slight yellowing of the concentrate may occur but will not effect potency. However, discard if markedly discolored.
- Do not discontinue without first talking with your doctor.

cholestyramine

Brand Names:
Questran (Bristol-Meyers Squibb)
Questran Light (Bristol-Meyers Squibb)

Generic Available: no

Type of Drug: antihyperlipidemic

Used for: Treatment of high blood cholesterol levels (hyperlipidemia), cardiovascular atherosclerosis, diarrhea associated with the bacteria *Clostridium difficile*, and itching caused by partial biliary obstruction.

How This Medication Works: Binds bile acids in the gastrointestinal tract, encouraging their excretion and causing the body to convert more cholesterol into bile acid.

Dosage Form and Strength:
- tablets (1 g)
- powder (4-g packets, or large container with measuring scoop)

Storage:
- room temperature
- tightly closed
- protected from humidity

Administration:
- Usually taken twice daily but can be taken up to 6 times daily.
- Mix the contents of 1 powder packet or 1 level scoopful in no less than ¼ cup of water or non-carbonated beverage, or mix with fluids or semi-solid foods such as applesauce, fluid soups, or pulpy fruits. Do not take powder dry.
- Take other drugs at least 1 hour before or 4 to 6 hours after taking cholestyramine.
- Take before meals.

Precautions:

Do not use if:
- you are allergic to cholestyramine or colestipol.
- you have complete biliary obstruction.

Talk to your doctor if:
- you notice an increase in your tendency to bleed (bleeding gums or rectum).
- you are taking warfarin, digoxin, gemfibrozil, piroxicam, propranolol, tetracycline, a thiazide diuretic (such as hydrochlorothiazide or chlorthalidone), or thyroid supplements (such as levothyroxine).

Side Effects:

Major:
- severe constipation

Minor:
- constipation
- belching
- abdominal distention/bloating
- flatulence
- headache
- nausea
- heartburn

Time Required for Drug to Take Effect: Takes about 1 month of therapy to lower total cholesterol levels.

Symptoms of Overdose:
- severe abdominal pain
- nausea and vomiting
- severe constipation

Special Notes:
- Taking cholestyramine powder in tomato juice or pulpy juices may help mask the "sandy" texture of the powder and increase palatability.
- Cholestyramine is not a cure and you may have to take this medication for a long time.
- Cholestyramine may interfere with the absorption of the fat-soluble vitamins (A, D, E, and K). Your doctor may wish you to take vitamin supplements.
- Drinking 6 to 8 full glasses of water every day will help decrease constipation.
- Constipation, flatulence, and heartburn may disappear with continued use.

cimetidine

Brand Name: Tagamet (SK Beecham)

Generic Available: yes

Type of Drug: gastrointestinal (histamine H_2 antagonist)

Used for: Treatment of excess acid production in the stomach, ulcers, and heartburn (gastroesophageal reflux disease [GERD]).

How This Medication Works: Blocks the binding of histamine to sites in the stomach that would cause acid secretion.

Dosage Form and Strength:
- tablets (200 mg, 300 mg, 400 mg, 800 mg)
- liquid (300 mg/5 mL)

Storage:
- room temperature
- protected from humidity

Administration:
- If you are taking multiple doses daily, take with or immediately after meals unless your doctor has different instructions.
- If you are only taking 1 dose daily, take it before bedtime unless your doctor says differently.
- If taking antacids, seperate doses of cimetidine and antacid by 2 hours.

Precautions:
Do not use if:
- you are allergic to cimetidine or other histamine H_2 antagonists such as ranitidine, famotidine, or nizatidine.

Talk to your doctor if:
- you have kidney or liver disease.
- you are taking any other medications, especially theophylline, anticoagulants (such as warfarin), antidepressants (such as amitriptyline or fluoxetine), antibiotics, phenytoin, or medications for heart disease or high blood pressure (hypertension).

Side Effects:
Major:
- skin rash, hives, or itching
- confusion or blurred vision
- irregular heartbeat
- fever, sore throat

- swelling of eyelids
- tightness in chest
- unusual bleeding or bruising

Minor:
- constipation or diarrhea
- decreased sexual ability or desire
- dizziness or drowsiness
- headache
- dry mouth
- increased sweating
- joint or muscle pain
- loss of appetite
- nausea or vomiting
- ringing or buzzing in the ears (tinnitus)
- swelling of breasts (in men and women)
- hair loss

Time Required for Drug to Take Effect: Starts to work within 1 to 2 hours, but ulcer healing may require 4 to 12 weeks of therapy.

Symptoms of Overdose:
- difficulty breathing
- irregular heartbeat
- tremors
- vomiting
- diarrhea
- light-headedness

Special Notes:
- Do not use any over-the-counter medications unless you check first with your physician and pharmacist.

- Avoid medications that may make your ulcer worse, including nonsteroidal anti-inflammatory drugs (aspirin, ibuprofen, naproxen, ketoprofen).
- If you are smoking, you should quit. If you continue to smoke, you should try not to smoke after the last dose of cimetidine for the day.
- This medication may cause drowsiness. Use caution when operating a motor vehicle or operating dangerous machinery.
- Avoid alcohol or other medications that may make you drowsy or dizzy, such as antihistamines, sedatives, tranquilizers, pain relievers, seizure medications, and muscle relaxants.
- Tell the doctor you are taking cimetidine if you are going to have a skin test for allergies.
- Tell the doctor or dentist you are taking cimetidine before undergoing any surgery or emergency treatment.

ciprofloxacin

Brand Name: Cipro (Miles)

Generic Available: no

Type of Drug: antibiotic

Used for: Treatment of infections of the ear, respiratory tract, skin, bone, and genitourinary tract.

How This Medication Works: Interferes with bacterial DNA gyrase, an enzyme vital for bacterial cell growth and reproduction.

Dosage Form and Strength: tablets (250 mg, 500 mg, 750 mg)

Storage:
- room temperature
- tightly closed
- protected from humidity

Administration:
- Usually taken twice daily.
- Take until completely gone, even if symptoms have improved.
- Take at even intervals, every 12 hours.
- May be taken without regard to meals.
- Take each dose with 6 to 8 ounces of water.
- Do not take antacids such as ferrous sulfate, zinc sulfate, or sucralfate for at least 2 hours before or 2 hours after ciprofloxacin dose.

Precautions:
Do not use if:
- you are allergic to ciprofloxacin or other drugs in the fluoroquinolone family, such as nalidixic acid or norfloxacin.
- medicine is beyond the expiration date.

Talk to your doctor if:
- you are taking probenecid, cimetidine, phenytoin, warfarin, theophylline, or cyclosporine.

Side Effects:
Major:
- hallucinations
- swelling of the tongue or lips
- rash

- shortness of breath
- severe diarrhea
- chest pain

Minor:
- restlessness
- nausea or stomach upset
- diarrhea

Time Required for Drug to Take Effect:

Begins to kill bacteria within hours of your first dose. However, you must continue to take ciprofloxacin for the full course of treatment, even if symptoms disappear.

Symptoms of Overdose:

- seizures
- renal failure

Special Notes:

- Avoid the use of caffeine while taking this drug.
- Do not use for infections other than the one for which it was prescribed.
- Discard liquid after 7 days (14 days, if refrigerated).
- Long-term treatment may lead to bacteria and fungus not sensitive to ciprofloxacin.
- Avoid excessive sunlight. Drugs in this class have caused extreme sensitivity to the sun, whether or not you wear a sunblock.

cisapride

Brand Name: Propulsid (Janssen)

Generic Available: no

Type of Drug: gastrointestinal stimulant

Used for: Treatment of diabetic stomach problems and heartburn (gastroesophageal reflux disease [GERD]).

How This Medication Works: Increases the release of acetylcholine, which increases the movement inside the stomach and intestines. Also strengthens the muscle between the esophagus and the stomach so food does not reflux, or back up.

Dosage Form and Strength: tablets (10 mg)

Storage:
- room temperature
- protected from humidity

Administration:
- Take at least 15 minutes before meals and/or at bedtime.

Precautions:
Do not use if:
- you are allergic to cisapride.

Talk to your doctor if:
- you have bleeding from stomach or intestines (bloody stools), disorders of stomach or intestines, Parkinson disease, epilepsy or seizures, kidney disease, or liver disease.
- you are taking any other medications, especially digoxin, anticholinergics (such as atropine), warfarin, diazepam, cimetidine, ranitidine, and medications that make you drowsy.

Side Effects:

Major:
- skin rash, hives, or itching
- irregular heartbeat
- seizures or convulsions
- fever or sore throat

Minor:
- diarrhea, cramping, or gas
- nausea
- headache
- dry mouth
- nervousness
- difficulty sleeping
- unusual bleeding or bruising
- difficulty breathing

Time Required for Drug to Take Effect: Starts to work within 30 to 60 minutes.

Symptoms of Overdose:
- irregular heartbeat
- diarrhea
- seizures or convulsions

Special Notes:
- Do not use any over-the-counter medications unless you check first with your physician and pharmacist.
- This medication may cause drowsiness. Use caution when operating a motor vehicle or operating dangerous machinery.
- Avoid alcohol or other medications that may make you drowsy or dizzy, such as antihista-

mines, sedatives, tranquilizers, pain relievers, seizure medications, and muscle relaxants.
- If you experience dryness of the mouth, try sugarless candy or gum, ice chips, or a saliva substitute.

clarithromycin

Brand Name: Biaxin (Abbott)

Generic Available: no

Type of Drug: antibiotic

Used for: Treatment of infections of the respiratory tract, skin, and genitourinary tract.

How This Medication Works: Inhibits protein synthesis in invading bacteria.

Dosage Form and Strength:
- tablets (250 mg, 500 mg)
- suspension (125 mg/5 mL, 250 mg/5 mL)

Storage:
- room temperature
- tightly closed
- protected from humidity

Administration:
- Usually taken twice daily.
- Take at even intervals, every 12 hours.
- May be taken without regard to meals.
- Shake suspension well before measuring dose.
- Take until completely gone, even if symptoms have improved.

Precautions:

Do not use if:
- you are allergic to clarithromycin or other drugs in the erythromycin family such as azithromycin.
- medicine is beyond the expiration date.

Talk to your doctor if:
- you are taking theophylline, zidovudine, digoxin, warfarin, carbamazepine, or terfenadine.

Side Effects:

Major:
- rash
- swelling of tongue or lips
- chest pain

Minor:
- diarrhea
- nausea or abdominal pain
- abnormal taste

Time Required for Drug to Take Effect:

Begins to kill infecting bacteria within hours after taking your first dose. However, you must continue to take clarithromycin for the full course of treatment, even if symptoms disappear.

Symptoms of Overdose:
- persistent nausea and vomiting
- severe diarrhea

Special Notes:
- Do not use for infections other than the one for which it was prescribed.
- Long-term treatment may lead to bacteria and fungus not sensitive to clarithromycin.

clonazepam

Brand Name: Klonopin (Roche)

Generic Available: no

Type of Drug: anticonvulsant

Used for: Treatment of seizures.

How This Medication Works: Enhances the activity of the neurotransmitter gamma amino butyric acid to depress the central nervous system.

Dosage Form and Strength: tablets (0.5 mg, 1 mg, 2 mg)

Storage:
- room temperature
- tightly closed

Administration:
- Usually taken 3 times daily.
- If you do miss a dose and it is within 1 hour, take the missed dose. Otherwise wait until next dose; do not double doses.
- Take with food if stomach upset occurs.

Precautions:

Do not use if:
- you are allergic to clonazepam or other drugs in the benzodiazepine family such as diazepam, lorazepam, and oxazepam.

Talk to your doctor if:
- you are taking other medications that depress the central nervous system including alcohol, pheno-

barbital, or narcotics (codeine, meperidine, morphine).
- you have asthma or other lung problems, kidney disease, or liver disease.
- you have been told that you snore.

Side Effects:
Major:
- confusion
- seizures
- hallucinations
- rash
- difficulty concentrating

Minor:
- unsteadiness
- drowsiness
- slurred speech or blurred vision

Time Required for Drug to Take Effect:
Controls seizures within 20 to 60 minutes; must be continued to maintain desired effect.

Symptoms of Overdose:
- continuing confusion or slurred speech
- severe weakness or drowsiness
- shortness of breath

Special Notes:
- This medication may cause drowsiness. Use caution when operating a motor vehicle or operating dangerous machinery.
- Do not drink alcohol while taking this medication.
- Do not discontinue without first talking with your doctor.

clonidine

Brand Names:
Catapres (Boehringer Ingelheim)
Catapres-TTS (Boehringer Ingelheim)

Generic Available:
- tablets: yes
- topical patch: no

Type of Drug: antihypertensive

Used for: Treatment of high blood pressure (hypertension), ulcerative colitis, pain after shingles, and diabetic diarrhea; suppression of withdrawal symptoms.

How This Medication Works: Acts on the central nervous system to dilate blood vessels.

Dosage Form and Strength:
- tablets (0.1 mg, 0.2 mg, 0.3 mg)
- topical patch (0.1 mg/24 hours, 0.2 mg/24 hours, 0.3 mg/24 hours)

Storage:
- room temperature
- tightly closed
- protected from humidity

Administration:
- Tablets are usually taken once or twice daily.
- Topical patches are applied every 5 to 7 days.
- Apply the patch to a hairless area of unbroken skin on the upper arm or torso, rotating sites with each patch.

Precautions:

Do not use if:
- you are allergic to clonidine or any of the components in the patch (such as the adhesive).

Talk to your doctor if:
- you have recently had a heart attack.
- you are taking a beta blocker (such as atenolol, metoprolol, or propranolol), or a tricyclic antidepressant (such as nortriptyline, amitriptyline, imipramine, or desipramine).
- you have heart disease or kidney disease.

Side Effects:

Major:
- generalized rash
- swelling of the mouth, lips, or tongue

Minor:
- drowsiness or dizziness
- dry mouth
- sedation
- constipation
- impotence or lack of sexual desire
- localized rash at site of patch application
- nightmares
- hair loss

Time Required for Drug to Take Effect:

Tablets lower blood pressure within 30 to 60 minutes; patches reach therapeutic blood levels in 2 to 3 days.

Symptoms of Overdose:

- severe sedation
- respiratory depression

- seizures
- low body temperature
- diarrhea

Special Notes:
- Do not discontinue without first talking with your doctor.
- Constipation, dizziness, headache, and fatigue will generally diminish after about 1 month of therapy.
- Use caution with alcohol consumption because clonidine may increase its effect.
- If you experience dryness of the mouth, try sugarless candy or gum, ice chips, or a saliva substitute.
- Tell the doctor or dentist you are taking this medication if you are going to have surgery or emergency treatment.
- Taking clonidine at bedtime (if prescribed once a day) will make the side effects of dizziness and sedation more tolerable.
- Clonidine is not a cure, and you may have to take this medication for a long time.

clotrimazole

Brand Names:
Lotrimin (Schering)
Mycelex (Miles)

Generic Available: yes

Type of Drug: topical antifungal

Used for: Treatment of fungal and yeast infections of the skin, such as ringworm, jock itch, and athlete's foot.

How This Medication Works: Prevents fungus and yeast from growing and reproducing.

Dosage Form and Strength:
- cream (1%)
- solution (1%)
- lotion (1%)

Storage:
- room temperature
- tightly closed
- protected from light

Administration:
- Clean affected area with soap and water, pat dry with a clean towel, and apply a thin layer to affected area twice daily or as directed.
- Do not bandage or cover unless directed by your doctor.
- Be sure to complete the prescribed course of therapy even if symptoms improve.
- If you miss a dose, apply the medication as soon as you remember. If it is time for the next dose, skip the missed dose; do not apply double the amount.

Precautions:
Do not use if:
- you are allergic to clotrimazole.

Talk to your doctor if:
- your condition has not improved in 4 weeks.

Side Effects:

Major:
- blistering, peeling, or irritation of the skin
- swelling

Minor:
- burning, itching, stinging, or redness

Time Required for Drug to Take Effect:

Improvement may not be noticeable for up to 1 week and may not resolve completely for up to 4 weeks. Continue to apply medication for the full course of treatment, even if symptoms disappear.

Symptoms of Overdose: Not a problem when used on the skin. If accidentally ingested, contact your doctor or a poison control center for instructions.

Special Notes:
- Do not use for infections other than the one for which it was prescribed.
- Do not use around the eyes.

clotrimazole and betamethasone combination

Brand Name: Lotrisone (Schering)

Generic Available: no

Type of Drug: topical antifungal with hormone

Used for: Treatment of fungal and yeast infections of the skin.

How This Medication Works: Prevents fungus and yeast from growing and reproducing and relieves skin inflammation, redness, swelling, and discomfort.

Dosage Form and Strength: cream (0.5% beta-methasone/1% clotrimazole)

Storage:
- room temperature
- tightly closed
- protected from light

Administration:
- Clean affected area with soap and water, pat dry with a clean towel, and apply a thin layer to affected area twice daily or as directed.
- Do not bandage or cover unless directed by your doctor.
- Be sure to complete the prescribed course of therapy even if symptoms improve.
- If you miss a dose, apply the medication as soon as you remember. If it is time for the next dose, skip the missed dose; do not apply double the amount.

Precautions:
Do not use if:
- you are allergic to clotrimazole, betamethasone, or any steroids.

Talk to your doctor if:
- you have blood vessel disease, cataracts, diabetes, fungal infections, glaucoma, shingles, stomach ulcers, skin infections, or tuberculosis.
- your condition has not improved in 4 weeks.

Side Effects:
Major:
- blistering, peeling, or irritation of the skin
- unexplained bruising
- increased hair growth
- loss of skin color
- swelling

Minor:
- acne
- burning, itching, or stinging
- dryness
- redness

Time Required for Drug to Take Effect:
Improvement may not be noticeable for up to 1 week and may not resolve completely for up to 4 weeks. Continue to apply medication for the full course of treatment, even if symptoms disappear.

Symptoms of Overdose: Not a problem when used on the skin. If accidentally ingested, contact your doctor or a poison control center for instructions.

Special Notes:
- Do not use for infections other than the one for which it was prescribed.
- Do not use around the eyes.

clozapine

Brand Name: Clozaril (Sandoz)

Generic Available: no

Type of Drug: antipsychotic

Used for: Treatment of schizophrenia or psychotic symptoms and sustained muscle contractions (dystonias) caused by Parkinson disease.

How This Medication Works: The exact mechanism of action of clozapine is unknown. However, it may block the neurotransmitter dopamine in the brain.

Dosage Form and Strength: tablets (25 mg, 100 mg)

Storage:
- room temperature
- tightly closed

Administration:
- Usually taken 1 to 2 times daily.
- Take first dose at bedtime, as significant sedation may occur when you first start taking clozapine.
- Your dosage is likely to be increased slowly.

Precautions:
Do not use if:
- you have had an allergic reaction to clozapine.

Talk to your doctor if:
- you are taking a medicine for high blood pressure, depression, seizures, insomnia, or anxiety.
- you are taking antihistamines, warfarin, digoxin, carbamazepine, phenytoin, or valproic acid.
- you have liver disease, kidney disease, an enlarged prostate, narrow angle glaucoma, a seizure disorder, heart disease, or high blood pressure (hypertension).

Side Effects:

Major:
- chest pain
- dizziness or fainting
- flu-like symptoms (fever, sore throat, malaise)

Minor:
- drowsiness, sedation
- excessive salivation
- vertigo
- constipation
- headache
- sweating
- nausea or vomiting
- heartburn
- weight gain

Time Required for Drug to Take Effect: Some
effects are seen within 15 minutes to 6 hours, but
optimal effect on schizophrenia may take 1 to 4 weeks.

Symptoms of Overdose:
- irregular heartbeat
- severe drowsiness, delirium, coma
- slowed or difficult breathing
- profound salivation

Special Notes:
- Clozapine can destroy the body's infection-fighting white blood cells (granulocytes). Therefore, if exposed to infection, your body is unable to defend itself and the infection can potentially be fatal. In view of the seriousness of this side effect, clozapine is reserved for people

who have not responded to the more traditional antipsychotics (haloperidol, thioridazine).

- Clozapine is available only through the Clozaril Patient Management System. The physician, laboratory, and pharmacist must all be registered in this system.
- You are required to have a blood test every 7 days to check your white blood cell count. Before dispensing clozapine, the pharmacist must first see the laboratory report to make sure your count has not fallen and then may dispense only a 1-week supply.
- Do not drink alcohol while taking this medication.
- Changing positions slowly when sitting and/or standing up may help decrease dizziness caused by this medication.
- If light-headedness or dizziness occurs it is important not to perform activities requiring mental alertness, such as driving a car or operating machinery.

codeine and acetaminophen combination

Brand Names:

Aceta with Codeine (Century)

Capital with Codeine (Carnrick)

Phenaphen-650 with Codeine (Robins)

Phenaphen with Codeine (Robins)

Tylenol with Codeine (McNeil)

Ty-tabs (Major)

Generic Available: yes

Type of Drug: analgesic

Used for: Relief of moderate to severe pain, suppression of cough, and treatment of diarrhea.

How This Medication Works: Codeine acts in the central nervous system to decrease the recognition of pain impulses. Acetaminophen works in the peripheral nervous system and blocks pain impulses.

Dosage Form and Strength:
- capsules (15 mg codeine/325 mg acetaminophen, 30 mg/325 mg, 60 mg/325 mg)
- oral elixir (12 mg/120 mg per 5 mL)
- tablets (7.5 mg/300 mg, 15 mg/300 mg, 30 mg/300 mg, 60 mg/300 mg, 30 mg/325 mg, 60 mg/325 mg, 30 mg/650 mg)

Storage:
- room temperature
- protected from humidity

Administration:
- Do not exceed the maximum number of doses per day. Never take more tablets per dose or more doses per day than your doctor has prescribed.
- Take with milk or food if stomach upset occurs.

Precautions:
Do not use if:
- you are allergic to codeine or other narcotics such as morphine or hydrocodone.
- you are allergic to acetaminophen.

Talk to your doctor if:
- you have alcoholism or other substance abuse problems; brain disease or head injury; colitis; seizures; emotional problems or mental illness; emphysema, asthma, or other lung diseases; kidney, liver, or thyroid disease; prostate problems or problems with urination; or gallbladder disease or gallstones.
- you are taking any other medications, especially those that can cause drowsiness such as antihistamines, barbiturates (phenobarbital), benzodiazepines (diazepam, alprazolam, lorazepam), muscle relaxants, and antidepressants.

Side Effects:
Major:
- skin rash or hives
- difficulty breathing
- fainting
- fast, slow, or pounding heart beat
- frequent urge to urinate
- painful or difficult urination
- hallucinations
- mental depression
- pinpoint red spots on body
- unusual bruising or bleeding
- trembling or uncontrolled muscle movements
- yellow eyes or skin (jaundice)

Minor:
- nausea
- constipation
- drowsiness
- dry mouth

- general discomfort or illness
- loss of appetite
- difficulty sleeping
- nervousness or restlessness

Time Required for Drug to Take Effect: Starts
to work within 30 to 60 minutes.

Symptoms of Overdose:
- cold, clammy skin
- severe confusion
- seizures
- diarrhea, and stomach cramps or pain
- severe dizziness, severe drowsiness
- low blood pressure, slowed heart beat
- protracted nausea or vomiting
- severe nervousness or restlessness
- pinpoint pupils of eyes
- shortness of breath or difficulty breathing

(Symptoms associated with acetaminophen may not occur until 2 to 4 days after the overdose is taken, but it is important to begin treatment as soon as possible after the overdose to prevent liver damage or death.)

Special Notes:
- This medication may cause drowsiness. Do not operate a motor vehicle or other machinery while you are taking this medication.
- Codeine, morphine, and other narcotics (oxy-codone, hydrocodone) cause constipation. This side effect may be diminished by drinking 6 to 8 full glasses of water each day. If using this med-

ication for chronic pain, adding a stool softener/laxative combination may be necessary.
- Check with your physician or pharmacist before using any over-the-counter medications.
- When codeine is used over a long period of time, your body may become tolerant and require larger doses.
- Do not stop taking this medication abruptly or you may experience unpleasant symptoms of withdrawal.
- Nausea and vomiting may occur, especially after the first few doses. This effect may go away if you lie down for a while.
- If you experience dryness of mouth, try sugarless candy or gum, ice chips, or a saliva substitute.
- Do not drink alcohol while taking this medication.

colchicine

Brand Names:
Colchicine (Abbott)
Colchicine (Lilly)

Generic Available: yes

Type of Drug: antigout

Used for: Prevention and treatment of gout.

How This Medication Works: Reduces the deposition of uric acid crystals.

Dosage Form and Strength: tablets (0.5 mg, 0.6 mg)

Storage:
- room temperature
- protected from humidity

Administration:
- Colchicine can be used during an acute attack or it may be taken on a long-term basis to prevent gout attacks. The instructions for using it during an acute attack are different from the instructions for using it on a long-term basis.
- May be taken with food or water if stomach upset occurs.

Precautions:
Do not use if:
- you are allergic to colchicine.

Talk to your doctor if:
- you drink alcohol or are taking any other medications, especially antibiotics and medications for diabetes, heart disease, cancer, depression, thyroid disease, or seizures.
- you have heart disease; blood diseases; diarrhea or other stomach or intestinal diseases; or kidney or liver disease.

Side Effects:
Major:
- skin rash, hives, or itching
- difficult or painful urination
- fever or sore throat
- muscle or stomach aches
- tingling in hands or feet
- unusual bleeding or bruising

- diarrhea
- nausea or vomiting

Minor:
- drowsiness
- loss of appetite
- hair loss

Time Required for Drug to Take Effect: Starts to work within 30 minutes to 2 hours.

Symptoms of Overdose:
- blood in urine or stool
- burning feeling in throat, stomach, or skin
- nausea, vomiting, or diarrhea
- fever
- mood changes
- muscle weakness
- difficulty breathing

Special Notes:
- Check with your physician or pharmacist before using any over-the-counter medications.
- Colchicine may cause drowsiness. Use caution when operating a motor vehicle or dangerous machinery.
- Do not drink alcohol when taking colchicine.

cromolyn

Brand Names:
Gastrocrom (Fisons)   Nasalcrom (Fisons)
Intal (Fisons)

Generic Available: no

Type of Drug: respiratory drug (antiasthma, antiallergic)

Used for: Prevention of allergy and asthma attacks.

How This Medication Works: Prevents certain cells (mast cells) from breaking down and releasing substances (histamine and SRS-A) which can cause wheezing, breathing difficulty, and an asthma attack.

Dosage Form and Strength:
- capsules (100 mg)
- capsules used with inhalation device (20 mg)
- inhaler (800 µg/inhalation)
- solution for nebulizer (10 mg/mL)
- solution, nasal (40 mg/mL)

Storage:
- room temperature
- protected from humidity

Administration:
- Have your doctor or pharmacist demonstrate the proper procedure for using your inhaler and practice your technique in front of them.
- Gargling and rinsing your mouth each time after you take cromolyn may help prevent dryness, hoarseness, and irritation of the throat and mouth.

Precautions:
Do not use if:
- you are allergic to cromolyn or nedocromil.

Talk to your doctor if:
- you have heart, kidney, or liver disease.
- you are taking any other medications.

Side Effects:

Major:
- skin rash, hives, or itching
- difficulty breathing
- difficulty urinating
- frequent urge to urinate
- dizziness
- headache
- joint pain or swelling
- nausea or vomiting
- swelling of the face, lips, eyelids, hands, feet, or inside the mouth
- chest pain
- chills or sweating
- difficulty swallowing
- muscle pain or weakness

Minor:
- cough
- dryness of the mouth or throat
- sneezing
- stuffy nose
- throat irritation or hoarseness
- watering eyes
- unpleasant taste

Time Required for Drug to Take Effect: Starts
working within minutes. However, it requires a period of 4 weeks of continuous cromolyn to achieve its maximal effectiveness.

Symptoms of Overdose:
- difficulty breathing or swollen throat
- painful urination

Special Notes:
- This medication is used to prevent asthma attacks. It is not useful once an acute asthma attack has begun. In fact, it may make the attack worse.
- Check with your physician and pharmacist before you use any over-the-counter medications.
- Be sure that you keep track of how many inhalations are left and get your medication refilled about 1 week before you expect to run out.
- One capsule form (Intal) is to be used with an inhalation device. The other capsules (Gastrocrom) are to be taken by mouth.
- Sometimes a spacer device is used with your inhaler. This device helps the medication get to the lungs instead of staying in the mouth or throat.

cyanocobalamin (vitamin B$_{12}$)

Brand Names:
Rubramin PC (Apothecon)
Betalin (Lilly)

Generic Available: yes

Type of Drug: blood modifier

Used for: Treatment of vitamin B$_{12}$–deficiency anemia (shortage of vitamin B$_{12}$).

How This Medication Works: Replaces vitamin B_{12} that is needed to make red blood cells.

Dosage Form and Strength: injection (100 µg/mL, 1000 µg/mL)

Storage:
- room temperature
- protected from light

Administration:
- Usual dose is 30 µg to 100 µg for 5 to 7 days, then 100 µg or 200 µg once per month.
- If you miss a dose, take the dose as soon as you remember; do not double up doses.

Precautions:

Do not take if:
- you have had a severe allergic or unusual reaction to cyanocobalamin, vitamin B_{12}, or cobalt.

Talk to your doctor if:
- you have rheumatoid arthritis, alcoholism, genetic disorders (such as homocystinuria or methylmalonic aciduria), liver disease, kidney disease, blood diseases, other forms of anemia, colitis, intestine problems, stomach disease, pancreatic disease, infections (acute or chronic, especially worms), or thyroid disease.

Side Effects:

Major:
- wheezing or difficulty breathing
- skin rash or itching after injection
- swelling of the mouth or throat

Minor:
- transient diarrhea
- pain at the site of injection

Time Required for Drug to Take Effect: Starts to replace deficiency almost immediately and may or may not have to be continued after vitamin B_{12} levels are restored, depending on the cause of the deficiency.

Symptoms of Overdose: polycythemia vera (blood disease)

Special Notes:
- Check with your doctor to see how long you need to take the medication.
- Check with your physician or pharmacist before using any over-the-counter medication.
- In some cases failure to continue life-long treatment will cause irreversible spinal cord damage and possible paralysis.
- Oral vitamin B_{12} is not effective in treatment of pernicious anemia.

cyclobenzaprine

Brand Name: Flexeril (Merck)

Generic Available: yes

Type of Drug: skeletal muscle relaxant

Used for: Relief of pain and muscle spasms due to muscle injury or osteoarthritis and treatment of fibromyalgia.

How This Medication Works: Acts within the brain to reduce muscle activity.

Dosage Form and Strength: tablets (10 mg)

Storage:
- room temperature
- tightly closed

Administration:
- Usually taken 3 times daily, approximately every 8 hours (sometimes less for elderly patients).

Precautions:
Do not use if:
- you have ever had an allergic reaction to cyclobenzaprine.
- you are taking (or have taken within 14 days) a monoamine oxidase (MAO) inhibitor such as phenelzine or tranylcypromine.

Talk to your doctor if:
- you have heart problems such as a recent heart attack, abnormal heart beat, or heart failure.
- you are taking an antidepressant, particularly a tricyclic antidepressant such as amitriptyline or imipramine.
- you have glaucoma, difficulty urinating, severe constipation, severe dry mouth, anxiety, or nervousness.

Side Effects:
Major:
- chest pain
- unusually high or low blood pressure

- fainting
- difficulty breathing
- dilated pupils
- severe confusion or hallucinations
- severe constipation
- difficulty urinating
- flulike symptoms
- swelling of face or tongue
- abnormal movements
- numbness in arms or legs
- unusual muscle stiffness or soreness

Minor:
- drowsiness
- dizziness
- fatigue
- blurred vision
- headache
- nervousness
- unpleasant taste
- sun sensitivity
- stomach upset
- bloating, gas

Time Required for Drug to Take Effect:
Begins working in approximately 1 hour.

Symptoms of Overdose:
- seizures
- coma
- unusual confusion or agitation
- hallucinations
- muscle rigidity
- vomiting

- severe constipation
- difficulty urinating
- dilated pupils
- fainting
- abnormal heart beat

Special Notes:

- This medicine is not usually recommended for more than 2 or 3 weeks.
- Do not drink alcohol while using this medicine.
- Use a sunblock with at least SPF 15 when outside because cyclobenzaprine may increase your sensitivity to the sun.

cyproheptadine

Brand Name: Periactin (Merck)

Generic Available: yes

Type of Drug: antihistamine

Used for: Treatment of allergies, hay fever, and hives.

How This Medication Works: Blocks histamine—a substance that causes sneezing, itching, and runny nose.

Dosage Form and Strength:

- tablets (4 mg)
- syrup (2 mg/5 mL)

Storage:

- room temperature
- protected from humidity

Administration:
- Take with full glass of water; drink plenty of fluids while taking cyproheptadine.
- Take with food if stomach upset occurs.

Precautions:
Do not use if:
- you are allergic to cyproheptadine or other antihistamines such as diphenhydramine, terfenadine, or hydroxyzine.

Talk to your doctor if:
- you have asthma, enlarged prostate, difficulty urinating, or glaucoma.
- you are taking any other medications, especially antidepressants or antibiotics.

Side Effects:
Major:
- skin rash, hives, or itching
- sore throat or fever
- hallucinations
- fainting, seizures, or convulsions
- difficulty breathing
- nervousness or restlessness

Minor:
- drowsiness, dizziness, or confusion
- thickening of mucous
- difficult or painful urination
- irregular heartbeat
- increased sensitivity to sun
- increased sweating
- increased appetite
- nightmares

Time Required for Drug to Take Effect: Starts to work within 90 to 120 minutes.

Symptoms of Overdose:
- dry mouth, throat, or nose
- flushed skin
- dilated pupils
- difficulty breathing
- dizziness or drowsiness
- excitation

Special Notes:
- Check with your physician and pharmacist before you use any over-the-counter medications.
- Tell the doctor you are taking cyproheptadine before you have a skin test for allergies.
- Do not drink alcohol or take other medications that cause drowsiness or mental slowing.
- This medication may cause drowsiness. Do not operate a motor vehicle or other machinery while you are taking this medication.
- If you experience dryness of the mouth, try sugarless candy or gum, ice chips, or a saliva substitute.
- Tell the doctor or dentist you are taking this medication if you are going to have surgery or emergency treatment.

dantrolene

Brand Name: Dantrium (Proctor & Gamble)

Generic Available: no

Type of Drug: muscle relaxant

Used for: Treatment of muscle spasticity caused by multiple sclerosis, spinal cord injury, cerebral palsy, or stroke.

How This Medication Works: Acts directly on skeletal muscle to decrease muscle contractions.

Dosage Form and Strength: capsules (25 mg, 50 mg, 100 mg)

Storage:
- room temperature
- tightly closed

Administration:
- Initial dose is usually 25 mg daily. Dose is slowly increased and may be given up to 3 or 4 times daily. The effective dose differs among patients.
- Capsules may be opened and the contents mixed with a small amount of fruit juice or other liquid.

Precautions:
Do not use if:
- you have ever had an allergic reaction to dantrolene.
- you have severe liver problems such as hepatitis or cirrhosis.

Talk to your doctor if:
- you are taking verapamil, warfarin, estrogens, high doses of acetaminophen, antibiotics, steroids, androgens (male hormones), or any medicines that cause drowsiness or dizziness.

- you are taking medicines for heart disease, respiratory disease (breathing problems), seizures, mental problems, or rheumatoid arthritis.

Side Effects:

Major:

- seizures
- chest pain
- painful or difficulty breathing
- stomach or abdominal pain or tenderness
- yellowing of the skin or eyes (jaundice)
- dark colored urine
- black, tarry stools
- skin rash or itching
- unusual difficulty urinating
- severe diarrhea
- chills and fever
- new swelling or pain in leg

Minor:

- drowsiness
- dizziness or light-headedness
- unusual weakness or tiredness
- blurred vision
- slurred speech
- unusual nervousness or confusion
- headache
- decreased appetite
- difficulty swallowing
- mild diarrhea

Time Required for Drug to Take Effect:

Begins to works in days to weeks (benefit should occur within 45 days).

Symptoms of Overdose:
- coma or extreme sedation
- vomiting
- seizures

Special Notes:
- Your doctor may order blood tests to monitor your liver function.
- Check with your physician or pharmacist before you use any over-the-counter medications.
- Do not drink alcohol when using this medicine.
- Use a sunblock with at least SPF 15 when outside because dantrolene may increase your sensitivity to the sun.

dexamethasone

Brand Names:
Decadron (Merck)
Dexone (Solvay)

Generic Available: yes

Type of Drug: hormone (adrenal cortical steroid)

Used for: Treatment of rheumatoid arthritis, lung diseases, lupus, ulcerative colitis, eye disorders, skin problems, poison ivy, and some cancers.

How This Medication Works: Dexamethasone is a cortisonelike substance naturally produced in the body. In most conditions it is unknown how it works but often the benefits are from decreasing inflammation.

Dosage Form and Strength:
- tablets (0.25 mg, 0.5 mg, 0.75 mg, 1 mg, 1.5 mg, 2 mg, 4 mg, 6 mg)
- elixir (0.5 mg/5 mL)
- solution (0.5 mg/5 mL, 0.5 mg/0.5 mL)

Storage:
- room temperature
- tightly closed
- protected from light

Administration:
- The dosage of dexamethasone varies from person to person depending on the disease being treated.
- If you are taking dexamethasone once daily, take it before 9:00 A.M.
- To prevent stomach upset, take it with food or milk.
- If you miss a dose and you are taking it more than once a day, take the dose as soon as you remember it; if you do not remember until the next dose, double the dose and return to your regular schedule. If you are taking the dose once a day, take the dose as soon as you remember it unless it is the next day; if it is the next day, do not double the dose, but take your regular dose, and return to your regular schedule. If you miss a dose taking it every other day, take the dose as soon as you remember it that day; if it is the day after the dose was to be taken, take it and start over on the every-other-day cycle skipping the next day and taking it the following day. If you miss more than one dose, call your doctor.

Precautions:

Do not use if:
- you have had an allergic reaction to dexamethasone, betamethasone, cortisone, prednisolone, prednisone, hydrocortisone, triamcinolone, or any other steroids.

Talk to your doctor if:
- you have bone disease, diabetes, emotional problems, glaucoma, fungal infections, heart disease, high blood pressure, high blood cholesterol levels, kidney disease, liver disease, myasthenia gravis, stomach problems (ulcers, gastritis), thyroid disease, tuberculosis, or ulcerative colitis.
- you are taking any medication, especially aspirin or nonsteroidal anti-inflammatory drugs (ibuprofen, indomethacin), anticoagulants (warfarin), cholestyramine, colestipol, diabetes medications (insulin, glipizide, tolbutamide), diuretics (hydrochlorothiazide, furosemide), seizure medications (phenobarbital, phenytoin), or tuberculosis medications (isoniazid, rifampin).

Side Effects:

Major:
- acne or other skin problems
- back or rib pain
- unusual, frequent, or severe bleeding or bruising
- bloody or black, tarry stools
- blurred vision
- eye pain
- fever
- headaches

- slow wound healing
- mood changes
- muscle weakness or wasting
- weight gain (3 to 5 pounds in a week)
- seizures
- shortness of breath
- sore throat
- stomach enlargement
- stomach pain
- thinning of the skin
- increased thirst
- increased urination

Minor:
- dizziness
- increased appetite
- indigestion
- increased sweating
- reddening of the skin on the face
- restlessness or sleep disorders

Time Required for Drug to Take Effect: Varies depending on the condition treated.

Symptoms of Overdose:
- agitation
- mania
- psychotic behavior

Special Notes:
- Dexamethasone can cause low potassium levels. Orange juice and bananas can replace some potassium. Talk to your doctor before making diet changes.

- If you take dexamethasone longer than a week, the dosage may need adjustments during stressful times. Tell your doctor if you have an infection or injury or if you have to have surgery.
- If you are taking dexamethasone for long periods of time, it may cause glaucoma and cataracts.
- Long-term dexamethasone therapy may increase your blood sugar and even cause diabetes.
- While you are taking dexamethasone you should not receive live vaccinations or immunizations.
- If you take the solution, it must be measured accurately with a dropper or special medication measuring spoon or cup. Do not use a kitchen spoon; the dose will not be accurate.

diazepam

Brand Names:
Valium (Roche)
Valrelease (Roche)

Generic Available: yes

Type of Drug: antianxiety

Used for: Treatment of anxiety.

How This Medication Works: Depresses the central nervous system.

Dosage Form and Strength:
- tablets (2 mg, 5 mg, 10 mg)
- extended-release capsules (15 mg)
- oral solution (5 mg/mL, 5 mg/5 mL)

Storage:
- room temperature
- tightly closed

Administration:
- Usually taken once daily (extended-release capsules) or 2 to 4 times daily (solution and tablets).
- Swallow extended-release capsules whole; do not chew or crush.
- Mix oral solution with a beverage (water or juice) or semi-solid foods such as applesauce.

Precautions:
Do not use if:
- you have ever had an allergic reaction to diazepam or any other drug in the benzodiazepine family such as alprazolam, clonazepam, or oxazepam.

Talk to your doctor if:
- you are taking any other medications, especially those that depress the central nervous system such as alcohol, phenobarbital, or narcotics (such as codeine, meperidine, and morphine).
- you have asthma or other lung problems, kidney disease, or liver disease.
- you have been told you snore.

Side Effects:
Major:
- confusion or difficulty concentrating
- seizures
- hallucinations
- rash

Minor:
- unsteadiness
- drowsiness
- slurred speech
- blurred vision

Time Required for Drug to Take Effect:
Begins to work within 2 hours.

Symptoms of Overdose:
- continuing or worsening confusion and/or slurred speech
- severe weakness or drowsiness
- shortness of breath

Special Notes:
- This medication may cause drowsiness. Use caution when operating a motor vehicle or operating dangerous machinery.
- Do not discontinue without first talking with your doctor.
- Do not drink alcohol while taking this medication.

diclofenac

Brand Names:
Cataflam (Ciba-Geigy)
Voltaren (Ciba-Geigy)

Generic Available: no

Type of Drug: nonsteroidal anti-inflammatory drug
(analgesic, anti-inflammatory, and antipyretic)

Used for: Relief of pain associated with rheumatoid arthritis, osteoarthritis, ankylosing spondylitis, surgery, headache, dental problems, muscle aches, orthopedic procedures, backache, athletic injuries, and miscellaneous aches and pains. Reduces fever.

How This Medication Works: Inhibits substances called prostaglandins that cause pain and inflammation. Treats a fever by increasing heat loss from the body.

Dosage Form and Strength:
- tablets (50 mg)
- delayed- or extended-release tablets (25 mg, 50 mg, 75 mg)

Storage:
- room temperature
- tightly closed
- protected from moisture and sunlight

Administration:
- Usually taken 2 to 3 times daily.
- Take with a full glass of water.
- Take with meals or milk if stomach upset occurs.
- Do not lie down for at least 30 minutes after taking this medicine.
- Swallow delayed- or extended-release tablets whole; do not break, crush, or chew.

Precautions:
Do not use if:
- you have ever had an allergic reaction to diclofenac or any other nonsteroidal anti-

inflammatory drug such as ibuprofen, indomethacin, piroxicam, or aspirin.
- medicine is beyond the expiration date or is
unusual in appearance.

Talk to your doctor if:
- you are taking aspirin, another nonsteroidal anti-
inflammatory drug (such as ibuprofen, indomethacin, or piroxicam), anticoagulants (such as
warfarin), a steroid (such as prednisone), lithium,
beta blockers (such as atenolol or propranolol),
diuretics (such as furosemide or hydrochlorothiazide), or methotrexate.
- you have peptic ulcer disease, bleeding from your
stomach or intestines, bleeding abnormalities,
ulcerative colitis, high blood pressure (hypertension), kidney disease, liver disease, heart disease,
asthma, or nasal polyps.
- you smoke tobacco or drink alcohol.

Side Effects:
Major:
- blood in stool, or dark, tarry stool
- persistent or severe stomach or abdominal pain
- vomiting blood
- blood in urine or dark, smokey-colored urine,
- difficulty urinating
- rash
- difficulty breathing
- swelling of the eyelids, throat, lips, or face
- vision or hearing changes
- unexplained sore throat or fever
- unusual bleeding or bruising
- irregular heartbeat

Minor:
- stomach upset
- gas or heartburn
- diarrhea or constipation
- swelling of hands or feet
- dizziness
- drowsiness
- headache
- increased sensitivity to the sun or ultraviolet light

Time Required for Drug to Take Effect: Starts to relieve pain within 1 to 3 hours. However, in arthritis, it may take 2 to 4 weeks to feel the full benefits.

Symptoms of Overdose:
- stomach pain or nausea
- heartburn
- vomiting
- drowsiness or confusion
- headache
- loss of consciousness

Special Notes:
- Contact your physician if pain or fever worsens during treatment.
- Drinking alcohol and/or smoking tobacco products may increase your risk of bleeding from the stomach or intestines while taking diclofenac.
- Diclofenac contains sodium, which may worsen heart failure, high blood pressure, or ankle edema.
- Use a sunblock with at least SPF 15 when outside because diclofenac may increase your sensitivity to the sun.

- Tell the doctor or dentist you are taking diclofenac if you are going to have surgery or emergency treatment.

dicyclomine

Brand Names:
Bemote (Everett)

Bentyl (Lakeside)

Byclomine (Major)

Di-Spaz (Vortech)

Generic Available: yes

Type of Drug: gastrointestinal (anticholinergic)

Used for: Treatment of disorders of the stomach and intestines such as irritable bowel syndrome and cramps.

How This Medication Works: Decreases the contraction of the muscles of the stomach and intestine, slowing the movement of stomach and intestinal contents.

Dosage Form and Strength:
- tablets (20 mg)
- capsules (10 mg, 20 mg)
- syrup (10 mg/5 mL)

Storage:
- room temperature
- protected from humidity

Administration:
- Take 30 minutes to 1 hour before meals.

- Do not take antacids within 1 hour of taking dicy-clomine.
- To measure the correct amount of syrup to take, use a measuring device that can measure in milli-liters (mL or ml). An ordinary teaspoon is not accurate enough.

Precautions:

Do not use if:

- you are allergic to dicyclomine or other anti-cholinergics such as atropine or clidinium.

Talk to your doctor if:

- you have glaucoma, heart disease, high blood pressure, hernia, kidney disease, liver disease, thyroid disease, myasthenia gravis, bladder disease, prostate disease, or ulcerative colitis.
- you drink alcohol.
- you are taking medications such as antidepres-sants, antacids, antidiarrheals, antifungals, potas-sium, or other anticholinergics (such as atropine or clidinium).

Side Effects:

Major:

- skin rash, hives, or itching
- confusion
- fainting
- eye pain or blurred vision
- difficulty urinating
- difficulty swallowing

Minor:

- drowsiness or dizziness
- constipation or bloated feeling

- headache
- increased sensitivity to bright light
- nausea or vomiting
- decreased sweating

Time Required for Drug to Take Effect: Starts to work within 1 to 2 hours.

Symptoms of Overdose:
- blurred vision
- drowsiness, dizziness, or confusion
- dryness of mouth, throat, or nose
- irregular heartbeat
- hallucinations
- fever or skin flushing
- excitement

Special Notes:
- This medication may cause drowsiness. Use caution when operating a motor vehicle or operating dangerous machinery.
- Check with your physician or pharmacist before using any over-the-counter medications.
- Do not drink alcohol while taking this medication.
- If you experience dryness of the mouth, try sugarless candy or gum, ice chips, or a saliva substitute.
- Dicyclomine decreases your body's ability to sweat. Be careful to avoid getting overheated by outdoor activities in the heat, saunas, or hot baths and showers.
- Tell the doctor or dentist you are taking dicyclomine if you are going to have surgery or emergency treatment.

digoxin

Brand Names:
Lanoxicaps (Burroughs Wellcome)
Lanoxin (Burroughs Wellcome)

Generic Available: yes

Type of Drug: cardiovascular (cardiac glycoside)

Used for: Treatment of congestive heart failure and abnormal heart rhythms such as atrial fibrillation.

How This Medication Works: Increases the ability of the heart muscle to pump blood and prevents part of the heart from beating abnormally.

Dosage Form and Strength:
- tablets (0.125 mg, 0.25 mg)
- capsules (0.05 mg, 0.1 mg, 0.2 mg)

Storage:
- room temperature
- protected from humidity

Administration:
- Take with water or food (excluding foods high in fiber) to minimize upset stomach.
- Take at the same time every day.
- Take at least 1 hour after or at least 2 hours before you take antacids.

Precautions:
Do not use if:
- you have ever had an allergic or unusual reaction to digoxin.

Talk to your doctor if:
- you have kidney disease or thyroid disease
- you are taking any other medicines, especially antacids, diuretics, antibiotics, and other medicines for the heart and blood pressure.

Side Effects:

Major:
- loss of appetite
- nausea and vomiting
- diarrhea
- vision disturbances
- dizziness, disorientation
- palpitations
- hallucinations

Minor:
- drowsiness
- headache
- muscle weakness
- tiredness
- slower heart rate
- enlarged breasts (in men and women)

Time Required for Drug to Take Effect: Starts to work within 1 to 2 hours. However, the drug must be taken on a regular basis to achieve constant levels in the blood.

Symptoms of Overdose:
- nausea, vomiting, and diarrhea
- blurred vision or yellow/green halos
- headache
- drowsiness, dizziness, disorientation
- weakness

Special Notes:

- Digoxin is not a cure and you may have to take this medication for a long time.
- Ask your doctor to tell you the range for a safe heart rate, but generally it is important to call your physician if your heart rate falls below 50 beats per minute.
- Side effects should disappear with continued use.
- Do not change brands of digoxin unless your physician and pharmacist have approved.
- Check with your physician or pharmacist before using any over-the-counter medications.
- You will need to have certain blood tests while you are taking digoxin.

diltiazem

Brand Names:

Cardizem (Marion Merrell Dow)

Cardizem CD (Marion Merrell Dow)

Cardizem SR (Marion Merrell Dow)

Dilacor XR (Rhone-Poulenc Rorer)

Tiazac (Forest)

Generic Available: yes

Type of Drug: cardiovascular (calcium channel blocker)

Used for: Treatment of angina and high blood pressure (hypertension).

How This Medication Works: Inhibits smooth-muscle contraction and causes dilation of the blood vessels.

Dosage Form and Strength:
- tablets (30 mg, 60 mg, 90 mg, 120 mg)
- extended-release capsules (120 mg, 180 mg, 240 mg, 300 mg, 360 mg)
- sustained-release capsules (60 mg, 90 mg, 120 mg)

Storage:
- room temperature
- protected from humidity

Administration:
- Swallow sustained-release capsules whole; do not crush or chew.
- Take at the same time every day.

Precautions:
Do not use if:
- you have ever had an allergic reaction to diltiazem or another calcium channel blocker such as nifedipine or verapamil.

Talk to your doctor if:
- you have heart, kidney, or liver disease, or problems with circulation or your blood vessels.
- you are taking any other medications, especially carbamazepine, cyclosporin, or warfarin.

Side Effects:
Major:
- bleeding or bruising, especially in the gum area
- skin rash, itching

- difficulty breathing
- slow heartbeat (less than 50 beats per minute)
- chest pressure or discomfort
- fainting
- swelling of feet or lower legs

Minor:
- low blood pressure (light-headedness, dizziness)
- headache
- sexual dysfunction
- flushing
- drowsiness
- nausea, constipation
- tiredness

Time Required for Drug to Take Effect: Starts
to work within 30 to 60 minutes. However, it takes at least 2 to 4 weeks to see the maximal response.

Symptoms of Overdose:
- nausea and vomiting
- weakness
- dizziness or drowsiness
- confusion or slurred speech
- palpitations
- loss of consciousness

Special Notes:
- Changing positions slowly when sitting and/or standing up may help decrease dizziness caused by this medication.
- If light-headedness occurs, it is important not to perform activities requiring mental alertness, such as driving a car or operating machinery.

- Check with your physician or pharmacist before using any over-the-counter medications.
- Diltiazem is not a cure and you may have to take this medication for a long time.
- Ask your doctor to tell you the range for a safe heart rate, but generally it is important to call your physician if your heart rate falls below 50 beats per minute.
- Be careful to avoid becoming dehydrated or over-heated. Avoid saunas and strenuous exercise in hot weather, and drink plenty of fluids.
- Do not drink alcohol while taking this medication.

diphenoxylate and atropine combination

Brand Names:

Logen (Goldline)
Lomanate (Various)

Lomotil (Searle)
Lonox (Geneva)

Generic Available: yes

Type of Drug: antidiarrheal

Used for: Treatment of diarrhea.

How This Medication Works: Slows down the movement of the intestines.

Dosage Form and Strength:

- tablets (2.5 mg diphenoxylate/0.025 mg atropine)
- liquid (2.5 mg/0.025 mg per 5 mL)

Storage:

- room temperature
- protected from humidity

Administration:

- Dosages vary greatly depending on the severity of diarrhea; never take more than the doctor has recommended.
- Take each dose with a full glass of water.

Precautions:

Do not use if:

- you are allergic to diphenoxylate or atropine.

Talk to your doctor if:

- you have alcohol or drug abuse problems, colitis, infectious diarrhea, emphysema, asthma, chronic bronchitis, difficulty urinating, prostate trouble, gallbladder disease, glaucoma, heart disease, high blood pressure, hernia, kidney disease, liver disease, thyroid disease, or myasthenia gravis.
- you are taking any other medications, especially naltrexone, other anticholinergics (such as dicy-clomine or clidinium), antibiotics, antihistamines, antidepressants, or medications that make you drowsy.

Side Effects:

Major:

- skin rash, hives, or itching
- shortness of breath
- bloating
- constipation
- loss of appetite

- stomach pain with nausea and vomiting
- blurred vision
- difficulty urinating
- drowsiness
- irregular heartbeat
- difficulty breathing
- flushing of skin

Minor:
- dizziness or light-headedness
- dryness of skin and mouth
- headache
- decreased sweating

Time Required for Drug to Take Effect: Starts to work within 45 to 60 minutes.

Symptoms of Overdose:
- drowsiness
- light-headedness or dizziness
- blurred vision
- flushing of skin
- small pupils

Special Notes:
- This medication may cause drowsiness. Use caution when operating a motor vehicle or operating dangerous machinery.
- Check with your physician or pharmacist before using any over-the-counter medications.
- Avoid alcohol and medications that may make you drowsy or dizzy, such as antihistamines, cold medications, sedatives, tranquilizers, seizure medications, and muscle relaxants.

- If you experience dryness of the mouth, try sugar-less candy or gum, ice chips, or a saliva substitute.
- It is important that you drink plenty of fluids if you have diarrhea so that you do not become dehydrated. Avoid physical activities in hot weather and saunas.
- Diphenoxylate is related to narcotics and may be habit-forming. To prevent abuse, atropine has been added to produce unpleasant side effects if larger than prescribed doses are taken.

dipyridamole

Brand Name: Persantine (Boehringer Ingelheim)

Generic Available: yes

Type of Drug: blood modifier

Used for: Prevention of thromboembolism (blood clots), myocardial reinfarction (repeat heart attacks), transient ischemic attacks, and strokes.

How This Medication Works: Decreases platelet stickiness to prevent clotting.

Dosage Form and Strength: tablets (25 mg, 50 mg, 75 mg, 100 mg)

Storage:
- room temperature
- tightly closed
- protected from light

Administration:
- Usually prescribed at 75 to 100 mg 4 times daily.
- Take with food or milk to decrease stomach upset.
- If you miss a dose you can take the dose as soon as you remember unless it is less than 4 hours before the next dose, in which case skip the missed dose and return to the regular schedule; do not double the dose.

Precautions:
Do not use if:
- you have had an allergic reaction to dipyrid-amole.

Talk to your doctor if:
- you have angina pectoris or low blood pressure (hypotension).
- you are taking any other medications, especially anticoagulants (such as heparin or warfarin), aspirin, nonsteroidal anti-inflammatory agents (such as ibuprofen or indomethacin), salicylates, valproate, or valproic acid.

Side Effects:
Major:
- angina (chest pain)
- bleeding
- unusual, frequent, or severe bruising
- high blood pressure (hypertension)
- irregular heartbeats
- low blood pressure
- lung pain
- migraines

Minor:
- diarrhea
- dizziness
- headache
- nausea
- stomach irritation and cramps
- vomiting

Time Required for Drug to Take Effect: Starts having significant effect in approximately 1 week.

Symptoms of Overdose:
- back pain (severe)
- unusual bruising or bleeding
- black, tarry stools or red blood in your stools
- unusual, frequent, or severe bruising
- coughing up blood
- decreased alertness
- dizziness
- headache (severe or persistent)
- joint pain or swelling
- paralysis
- speech difficulty
- stomach pain or bloating
- urine changes (bloody, pink, or red tinged)
- unusual tiredness or weakness
- unsteadiness on your feet

Special Notes:
- The Food and Drug Administration (FDA) has determined that there is evidence that dipyridamole does not improve chronic angina, and it is usually replaced with more effective medications.

doxepin

Brand Names:
Adapin (Fisons)
Sinequan (Roerig)

Generic Available: yes

Type of Drug: tricyclic antidepressant

Used for: Treatment of depression, anxiety, chronic pain, itching with hives, and peptic ulcer disease.

How This Medication Works: Increases the action of the neurotransmitters norepinephrine and serotonin in the brain.

Dosage Form and Strength:
- capsules (10 mg, 25 mg, 50 mg, 75 mg, 100 mg, 150 mg)
- liquid/oral concentrate (10 mg/mL)

Storage:
- room temperature
- tightly closed

Administration:
- Usually taken at bedtime.
- May also be prescribed 2 to 3 times daily, depending on your response to the medicine.
- Can be taken without regard to food.
- Use dropper to measure dose of liquid medication.
- Drops should be mixed with one-half glass of water, milk, or citrus juices just before taking.

Precautions:

Do not use if:
- you have had an allergic reaction to doxepin or any other tricyclic antidepressant such as amitriptyline, clomipramine, and imipramine.
- you are taking an antidepressant of the monoamine oxidase (MAO) inhibitor type such as phenelzine and tranylcypromine.

Talk to your doctor if:
- you have glaucoma (angle closure type), heart disease, urinary or prostate problems, severe constipation, breathing problems, seizures, diabetes, or thyroid problems.
- you are taking cimetidine, clonidine, methyldopa, reserpine, guanethidine, sedatives, muscle relaxants, cold medications, antihistamines, decongestants, or stimulants.
- you use alcohol on a regular or occasional basis.

Side Effects:

Major:
- dizziness, confusion, or falls
- fainting
- rapid heartbeat
- chest pain
- severe constipation
- urinary retention
- rash
- severe sedation
- fever
- hallucinations
- restlessness or agitation
- severe sunburn

<u>*Minor:*</u>
- drowsiness
- dry mouth
- mild constipation
- weight gain
- unpleasant taste
- stomach upset

Time Required for Drug to Take Effect: The full therapeutic benefit of this medicine may take from 4 to 8 weeks.

Symptoms of Overdose:
- confusion
- hallucinations
- seizures
- extreme sedation
- very slow or rapid heartbeat
- low blood pressure
- difficulty breathing
- inability to urinate
- severe constipation
- dilated pupils

Special Notes:
- Know which "target symptoms" (restlessness, worry, fear, or changes in sleep or appetite) you are being treated for and be prepared to tell your doctor if your target symptoms are improving, worsening, or unchanged.
- Your doctor may order a blood test to make dose adjustments.
- Check with your physician or pharmacist before using any over-the-counter medications.

- Do not discontinue without first talking with your doctor.
- Never increase your dose without the advice of your doctor.
- If you have diabetes, you may notice a change in your blood sugar level when using this medicine.
- Use a sunblock with at least SPF 15 when outside because doxepin may increase your sensitivity to the sun.
- Once the medicine takes effect, your doctor may continue this medicine for a long period of time to maintain the antidepressant benefits.

doxycycline

Brand Names:
Vibra-Tabs (Pfizer)   Doryx (Parke-Davis)
Vibramycin (Pfizer)

Generic Available: yes

Type of Drug: antibiotic

Used for: Treatment of bacterial and fungal infections of the ear, respiratory tract, skin, genitourinary tract, and bone; prevention of traveler's diarrhea.

How This Medication Works: Inhibits protein synthesis in invading bacteria.

Dosage Form and Strength:
- tablets (50 mg, 100 mg)
- capsules (50 mg, 100 mg)
- syrup (50 mg/5 mL)

Storage:
- room temperature
- tightly closed
- protected from humidity

Administration:
- Usually taken once daily (every 12 hours for more severe infections).
- Take at even intervals.
- May be taken with food or milk.
- Avoid taking within 2 hours of antacids or iron preparations.

Precautions:
Do not use if:
- you are allergic to doxycycline or drugs in the tetracycline family.
- medicine is beyond the expiration date.

Talk to your doctor if:
- you are taking warfarin, carbamazepine, phenobarbital, phenytoin, cimetidine, digoxin, insulin, iron, lithium, or other antibiotics.

Side Effects:
Major:
- headache
- blurred vision
- rash
- swelling of tongue or lips
- unexplained muscle aches
- severe, persistent diarrhea

Minor:
- nausea or stomach upset
- diarrhea

Time Required for Drug to Take Effect:

Begins to kill infecting bacteria within hours after taking your first dose. However, you must continue to take doxycycline for the full course of treatment, even if symptoms disappear.

Symptoms of Overdose:

- loss of appetite
- severe nausea and vomiting

Special Notes:

- Use a sunblock with at least SPF 15 when outside because doxycycline may increase your sensitivity to the sun.
- Take until completely gone, even if symptoms have improved.
- Do not use for infections other than the one for which it was prescribed.
- Long-term treatment may lead to bacteria and fungus not sensitive to doxycycline.
- Doxycycline may decrease your need for insulin. Monitor blood glucose levels at least 4 times daily while on doxycycline.

enalapril

Brand Name: Vasotec (Merck)

Generic Available: no

Type of Drug: antihypertensive (angiotensin-converting enzyme [ACE] inhibitor)

Used for: Treatment of high blood pressure (hypertension), congestive heart failure, and kidney disease caused by diabetes (diabetic nephropathy), and preservation of heart function after a heart attack.

How This Medication Works: Inhibits an enzyme needed to make angiotensin. Angiotensin causes powerful constriction of blood vessels.

Dosage Form and Strength: tablets (2.5 mg, 5 mg, 10 mg, 20 mg)

Storage:
- room temperature
- tightly closed
- protected from humidity

Administration:
- Usually taken once or twice daily.
- May be taken without regard to food.

Precautions:
Do not use if:
- you are allergic to enalapril or other ACE inhibitors such as captopril or lisinopril.
- you have liver disease (bilateral renal artery stenosis).

Talk to your doctor if:
- you are taking a diuretic (such as hydrochlorothiazide or furosemide) or a potassium supplement.
- you are taking indomethacin, any nonsteroidal anti-inflammatory drug (such as aspirin, ibuprofen, naproxen, piroxicam, and ketoprofen), allopurinol, digoxin, lithium, or rifampin.

Side Effects:

Major:
- swelling of the mouth, lips, or tongue
- fainting
- generalized rash
- chest pain
- irregular heartbeat

Minor:
- cough
- headache
- dizziness
- fatigue
- impotence or decreased sexual desire

Time Required for Drug to Take Effect:

Usually starts to work after about 1 week of therapy, but sometimes several weeks of therapy are needed for enalapril to reach its maximum effect.

Symptoms of Overdose:

- very low blood pressure (dizziness, fainting)
- profound muscle weakness
- nausea, vomiting, and diarrhea

Special Notes:

- Avoid salt substitutes containing potassium.
- You will need laboratory blood work while on enalapril to monitor kidney function and electrolytes (sodium, potassium) in the blood.
- Avoid the use of aspirin or other nonsteroidal anti-inflammatory drugs such as ibuprofen, naproxen, and ketoprofen. Use acetaminophen for pain relief.

- Enalapril may cause a dry cough. Talk to your doctor if you develop a particularly bothersome cough.
- Use a sunblock with at least SPF 15 when outside because enalapril may increase your sensitivity to the sun.

erythromycin

Brand Names:

E-Mycin (Boots)
Ery-Tab (Abbott)

PCE Dispertab (Abbott)
Eryc (Parke-Davis)

Generic Available: yes

Type of Drug: antibiotic

Used for: Treatment of infections of the respiratory tract, skin, and genitourinary tract.

How This Medication Works: Inhibits protein synthesis in invading bacteria.

Dosage Form and Strength:

- tablets (250 mg, 333 mg, 500 mg)
- capsules (250 mg)

Storage:

- room temperature
- tightly closed
- protected from humidity

Administration:

- Usually taken 4 times daily.

- Take on an empty stomach, 1 hour before or 2 hours after a meal. (Enteric-coated capsules may be taken without regard to food.)
- Take at even intervals, every 6 hours.

Precautions:

Do not use if:

- you are allergic to erythromycin or drugs in the erythromycin family such as azithromycin or clarithromycin.
- medicine is beyond the expiration date.

Talk to your doctor if:

- you are taking any other medication, especially warfarin, astemizole, terfenadine, bromocriptine, carbamazepine, cyclosporine, digoxin, disopyramide, methylprednisolone, theophylline, triazolam, or other antibiotics.

Side Effects:

Major:

- rash
- swelling of tongue or lips
- chest pain

Minor:

- diarrhea or flatulence
- nausea or abdominal pain
- abnormal taste

Time Required for Drug to Take Effect:

Begins to kill infecting bacteria within hours after taking your first dose. However, you must continue to take erythromycin for the full course of treatment, even if symptoms disappear.

Symptoms of Overdose:
- severe nausea and vomiting
- persistent, severe diarrhea

Special Notes:
- Take until gone, even if symptoms improve.
- Do not use for infections other than the one for which it was prescribed.

estradiol (topical)

Brand Names:
Climara (Berlex)   Vivelle (Ciba-Geigy)
Estraderm (Ciba-Geigy)

Generic Available: no

Type of Drug: hormone

Used for: Controlling menopausal symptoms or prevention of osteoporosis in women.

How This Medication Works: Replaces estrogen losses that occur after menopause or ovary removal.

Dosage Form and Strength: patch (0.05 mg/24 hours, 0.1 mg/24 hours)

Storage:
- room temperature (below 86°F)
- in the original sealed pouches

Administration:
- Patches are applied once or twice a week; follow directions from your doctor.

- Read directions for application closely; they may vary between products.
- Wash and dry hands thoroughly before and after applying patch.
- Apply to a clean, dry, non-oily, and hairless area of the abdomen. (Another possible area is on the buttocks, but the abdomen is preferred.)
- Do not apply on cuts or abrasions.
- Press the disk firmly in place with your palm for 10 seconds, making sure there is good contact, especially around the edges.
- Do not put the patch on the same exact place each time; rotate patch placement so that you have at least 1 week in between repeating the patch in the same area.
- If you miss a dose, replace the patch as soon as you remember it; if it is time for the next dose, skip the missed dose; do not put on 2 patches.

Precautions:
Do not use if:

- you are allergic to estradiol, chlorotrianisene, conjugated estrogens, diethylstilbestrol, esterified estrogens, estrone estropipate, ethinyl estradiol, quinestrol, or the adhesive of the patch.
- you have breast cancer or abnormal vaginal bleeding.

Talk to your doctor if:

- you have endometriosis, gall bladder disease, high blood calcium levels from metastatic breast cancer, liver disease, or thrombophlebitis (blood clots).

- you are taking any other medication, especially bromocriptine, cyclosporine, dantrolene, or tamoxifen.

Side Effects:

Major:
- breast pain, tenderness, or enlargement
- breast tumors
- gall bladder disease
- leg or foot swelling (edema)
- involuntary muscular movements
- menstrual changes
- yellowing of the eyes and skin (jaundice)

Minor:
- decreased appetite
- contact lens problems
- diarrhea
- dizziness
- gum changes (tenderness, swelling, or pain)
- libido changes
- migraine headaches
- nausea
- skin irritation and redness
- stomach cramping or bloating

Time Required for Drug to Take Effect: Varies
depending on the type of condition treated.

Symptoms of Overdose: No acute problems have
been reported with estrogen overdoses.

Special Notes:
- Do not apply to breasts, waistline, or any area where clothing is tight fitting.

- Women with an intact uterus should not use estrogens alone; talk to your doctor about taking progestins to prevent endometrial cancer.
- If you are switching from oral estrogen to the patch, you should wait 1 week after stopping the pills before starting the patch.
- If the patch loosens or falls off, you may reapply the old patch or put on a new one.
- Regular brushing and flossing is necessary to help prevent gum side effects.

estrogens, conjugated (systemic)

Brand Name: Premarin (Wyeth-Ayerst)

Generic Available: yes

Type of Drug: hormone

Used for: Controlling menopausal symptoms and preventing osteoporosis in women; controlling prostate cancer in men.

How This Medication Works: Replaces estrogen losses that occur after menopause or ovary removal.

Dosage Form and Strength: tablets (0.3 mg, 0.625 mg, 1.25 mg, 2.5 mg)

Storage:
- room temperature
- tightly closed
- protected from light

Administration:
- Usually 0.3 mg to 1.25 mg daily for menopausal symptoms and estrogen replacement.
- Usually 1.25 mg to 2.5 mg 3 times daily for prostate cancer.

Precautions:
Do not use if:
- you are allergic to estradiol, chlorotrianisene, conjugated estrogens, diethylstilbestrol, esterified estrogens, estrone estropipate, ethinyl estradiol, or quinestrol.
- you have breast cancer or experience abnormal vaginal bleeding.

Talk to your doctor if:
- you have endometriosis, gall bladder disease, liver disease, thrombophlebitis (blood clots), or high blood calcium levels from metastatic breast cancer.
- you are taking any other medication, especially bromocriptine, cyclosporine, dantrolene, or tamoxifen.

Side Effects:
Major:
- breast pain or tenderness
- breast enlargement
- breast tumors
- gall bladder disease
- leg or feet swelling (edema)
- involuntary muscular movements
- menstrual changes
- yellowing of the eyes and skin (jaundice)

Minor:
- decreased appetite
- contact lens problems
- diarrhea
- dizziness
- gum changes (tenderness, swelling, or pain)
- increased libido in women; decreased in men
- migraine headaches
- nausea
- stomach cramping or bloating

Time Required for Drug to Take Effect: Varies depending on the type of condition treated.

Symptoms of Overdose: No acute problems have been reported with estrogen overdoses.

Special Notes:
- Women with an intact uterus should not use estrogens alone; talk to your doctor about taking progestins to prevent endometrial cancer.
- Regular brushing and flossing are necessary to help prevent gum side effects.
- For combinations of estrogen and medroxyprogesterone, see the medroxyprogesterone profile.

etodolac

Brand Name: Lodine (Wyeth-Ayerst)

Generic Available: no

Type of Drug: nonsteroidal anti-inflammatory drug (analgesic, anti-inflammatory, and antipyretic)

Used for: Treatment of osteoarthritis and pain.

How This Medication Works: Inhibits substances called prostaglandins that cause pain and inflammation.

Dosage Form and Strength:
- capsule (200 mg, 300 mg)
- tablet (400 mg)

Storage:
- room temperature
- tightly closed
- protected from moisture and light

Administration:
- Usually taken 2 to 4 times daily.
- Take with meals or milk if stomach upset occurs.
- If using antacids, separate doses of etodolac and antacid by 2 hours.
- Do not lie down for at least 30 minutes after taking this medicine.
- Take with a full glass of water (6 to 8 ounces).

Precautions:
Do not use if:
- you are allergic to etodolac or any other nonsteroidal anti-inflammatory drug such as ibuprofen, indomethacin, piroxicam, or aspirin.
- medicine is beyond the expiration date or unusual in appearance.

Talk to your doctor if:
- you are taking aspirin; another nonsteroidal anti-inflammatory drug such as ibuprofen, indomethacin, or piroxicam; anticoagulants such as warfarin;

steroids such as prednisone; lithium; diuretics such as furosemide or hydrochlorothiazide; or methotrexate.

- you have peptic ulcer disease, bleeding from your stomach or intestines, bleeding abnormalities, ulcerative colitis, high blood pressure (hypertension), kidney disease, liver disease, heart disease, asthma, or nasal polyps.
- you smoke tobacco or drink alcohol.

Side Effects:

Major:

- blood in stool, or dark, tarry stool
- persistent or severe stomach or abdominal pain
- vomiting blood
- blood in urine or dark, smokey-colored urine
- difficulty urinating
- rash
- difficulty breathing
- swelling of the eyelids, throat, lips, or face (allergic reaction)
- vision or hearing changes
- unexplained sore throat or fever
- unusual bleeding or bruising
- irregular heartbeat

Minor:

- stomach upset
- gas or heartburn
- diarrhea or constipation
- swelling of hands or feet
- dizziness or drowsiness
- headache
- increased sensitivity to the sun or ultraviolet light

Time Required for Drug to Take Effect: Starts to relieve pain in 1 to 3 hours. However, it may take 2 to 4 weeks to feel the full benefits of this medicine when treating arthritis.

Symptoms of Overdose:
- stomach pain or nausea
- heartburn
- vomiting
- drowsiness or confusion
- loss of consciousness
- headache

Special Notes:
- Drinking alcohol or smoking tobacco may increase your risk of bleeding from the stomach or intestines while taking etodolac.
- Use a sunblock with at least SPF 15 when outside because etodolac may increase your sensitivity to the sun.
- Tell the doctor or dentist you are taking etodolac if you are going to have surgery or emergency treatment.
- Contact physician if pain worsens during treatment.

famotidine

Brand Name: Pepcid (Merck)

Generic Available: no

Type of Drug: gastrointestinal (histamine H_2 antagonist)

Used for: Treatment of excess acid production in the stomach, ulcers, and heartburn (gastroesophageal reflux disease [GERD]).

How This Medication Works: Blocks the binding of histamine to sites in the stomach that would cause acid secretion.

Dosage Form and Strength:
- tablets (20 mg, 40 mg)
- suspension (40 mg/5 mL)

Storage:
- room temperature
- protected from humidity

Administration:
- If you are taking multiple doses daily, take with or immediately after meals unless your doctor has different instructions.
- If you are only taking 1 dose daily, take it before bedtime unless your doctor says differently.
- If using antacids, separate doses of famotidine and antacid by 2 hours.
- Shake the suspension well before measuring dose.

Precautions:
Do not use if:
- you are allergic to famotidine or other histamine H_2 antagonists such as cimetidine or ranitidine.

Talk to your doctor if:
- you have kidney or liver disease.
- you are taking any other medications, especially theophylline, anticoagulants (such as warfarin), antidepressants (such as amitriptyline, fluoxetine,

or trazodone), antibiotics, phenytoin, or medications for heart disease or high blood pressure (hypertension).

Side Effects:
Major:
- skin rash, hives, or itching
- confusion or blurred vision
- irregular heartbeat
- fever or sore throat
- swelling of eyelids
- tightness in chest
- unusual bleeding or bruising

Minor:
- constipation or diarrhea
- decreased sexual ability or desire
- dizziness or drowsiness
- headache
- dry mouth
- increased sweating
- joint or muscle pain
- loss of appetite
- nausea or vomiting
- ringing or buzzing in the ears (tinnitus)
- swelling of breasts (in men and women)
- hair loss

Time Required for Drug to Take Effect: Starts
to work within 1 hour. However, ulcer healing may require 4 to 12 weeks of therapy.

Symptoms of Overdose:
- difficulty breathing
- irregular heartbeat

- tremors
- vomiting
- diarrhea
- light-headedness

Special Notes:
- Check with your physician or pharmacist before taking any over-the-counter medications.
- Avoid medications that may make your ulcer worse, including nonsteroidal anti-inflammatory drugs (aspirin, ibuprofen, naproxen, ketoprofen).
- If you smoke, you should quit. If you continue, do not to smoke after the last dose of the day.
- This medication may cause drowsiness. Use caution when operating a motor vehicle or operating dangerous machinery.
- Avoid alcohol or drugs that may make you drowsy, such as antihistamines, sedatives, pain relievers, seizure medications, and muscle relaxants.
- Tell the doctor you are taking famotidine if you are going to have a skin test for allergies.
- If you experience dryness of the mouth, try sugarless candy or gum, ice chips, or a saliva substitute.
- Tell the doctor or dentist you are taking famotidine before undergoing any treatment.

felodipine

Brand Name: Plendil (Merck)

Generic Available: no

Type of Drug: calcium channel blocker

- Check with your physician or pharmacist before using any over-the-counter medications.
- Avoid becoming dehydrated or overheated. Avoid saunas and strenuous exercise in hot weather. Drink plenty of fluids.
- Do not drink alcohol while taking this medication.

fentanyl

Brand Names:

Duragesic–25 (Janssen)   Duragesic–75 (Janssen)
Duragesic–50 (Janssen)   Duragesic–100 (Janssen)

Generic Available: no

Type of Drug: analgesic

Used for: Relief of stable, chronic pain.

How This Medication Works: Decreases the central nervous system's recognition of pain impulses.

Dosage Form and Strength: patch (25 µg/hr, 50 µg/hr, 75 µg/hr, 100 µg/hr)

Storage:
- room temperature
- protected from humidity

Administration:
- Generally prescribed as 1 patch every 3 days (72 hours); in certain circumstances may be applied every 2 days (48 hours).
- Read directions for application closely; they may vary between products.

- Wash and dry hands thoroughly before and after applying patch.
- Apply to a clean, dry, non-oily area of the chest, upper back, or upper arms that is free of hair (clip hair, do not shave).
- Try to avoid areas that will be subject to the movement of your arms.
- Do not apply on cuts or abrasions.
- Do not put the patch on the same exact place each time; rotate patch placement so that you have at least 1 week in between repeating the patch in the same area.
- Remove the old (used) patch before applying the new one.
- Do not use soap, lotions, oils, or alcohol before applying a patch; they may irritate the skin or change the absorption of the drug.
- Apply patch to a prepared site immediately after removing from its sealed package.
- Press in place with the palm of your hand and hold firmly 10 to 20 seconds, making sure the edges of the patch adhere to the skin.
- Discard used patches carefully; they still contain a rather large reservoir of fentanyl. Fold the patch in half so that the adhesive section sticks to itself. Flush down the toilet as soon as possible after removal from your skin.

Precautions:
Do not use if:
- you are allergic to fentanyl or any related medications such as meperidine, diphenoxylate, or loperamide.

Talk to your doctor if:
- you have substance abuse problems or alcoholism; brain disease or head injury; colitis; seizures; emotional problems or mental illness; emphysema, asthma, or other lung diseases; kidney, liver, or thyroid disease; prostate problems or problems with urination; or gallbladder disease or gallstones.
- you have ever had an abnormal heart beat.
- you are taking any other medications, especially naltrexone, zidovudine, or medications that can cause drowsiness such as antihistamines, barbiturates (phenobarbital), benzodiazepines (diazepam, alprazolam, lorazepam), muscle relaxants, or antidepressants.

Side Effects:
Major:
- skin rash or hives
- severe confusion
- fainting
- seizures
- painful or difficult urination
- frequent urge to urinate
- fast, slow, or pounding heartbeat
- hallucinations
- irregular breathing or difficulty breathing
- depression
- trembling or uncontrolled muscle movements

Minor:
- constipation
- drowsiness
- dry mouth

- general feeling of discomfort or illness
- loss of appetite
- difficulty sleeping
- nervousness or restlessness

Time Required for Drug to Take Effect: Starts
to work within several hours. However, it takes at least
24 hours to reach maximum pain relief. It may take up
to 6 days after a dosage increase to feel the full pain-
relieving effect of the higher dose.

Symptoms of Overdose:
- cold, clammy skin
- severe confusion
- seizures
- diarrhea or stomach cramps
- severe dizziness or drowsiness
- continued nausea or vomiting
- severe nervousness or restlessness
- difficulty breathing
- slowed heartbeat

Special Notes:
- Do not operate a motor vehicle or other
  machinery while you are taking this medication.
- Fentanyl may cause constipation. This side effect
  may be diminished by drinking 6 to 8 full glasses
  of water each day. Increase fresh fruit in your diet.
  If using this medication for chronic pain, ask your
  doctor about adding a stool softener/laxative
  combination.
- Check with your physician or pharmacist before
  using any over-the-counter medications.

- When fentanyl is used over a long period, your body may become tolerant and require larger doses. If your pain is no longer relieved by the current dose, talk to your doctor or pharmacist.
- Do not stop taking this medication abruptly.
- Nausea and vomiting may occur, especially after the first few doses; this effect will generally diminish with time.
- Do not drink alcohol while taking this medication.
- If you experience dry mouth, try sugarless candy, or gum, ice chips, or a saliva substitute.
- If you think you or anyone else may have taken an overdose, get emergency help immediately.
- Transdermal (skin) patches should not be used for acute pain relief.
- Use this medication as prescribed; do not exceed the dose or frequency prescribed by your doctor.
- Keep away from children and pets.

ferrous sulfate

Brand Names:

Feosol (SK Beecham)
Fer-In-Sol Syrup (Mead
  Johnson)
Fero-Gradumet (Abbott)

Mol-Iron (Schering-
  Plough)

Generic Available: yes

Type of Drug: blood modifier

Used for: Treatment of iron-deficiency anemia.

How This Medication Works: Replaces iron that is needed to make the oxygen-carrying hemoglobin in red blood cells.

Dosage Form and Strength:
- tablets (195 mg, 300 mg, 325 mg)
- enteric-coated tablets (300 mg, 325 mg)
- extended-release tablets (525 mg)
- extended-release capsules (150 mg, 250 mg)
- elixir (220 mg/5 mL)
- solution (90 mg/5 mL)
- capsules (300 mg)

Storage:
Tablets and capsules:
- room temperature
- tightly closed
- protected from light

Elixir and solution:
- refrigerated (do not freeze)
- tightly closed
- protected from light

Administration:
- Usual dosage is 1 capsule or tablet (160 to 324 mg) 3 or 4 times daily.
- If you miss a dose for 1 or more days, just resume your prescribed schedule when you remember; do not double the dose.
- Do not crush tablets or capsules.
- For liquids, mix with water or juice and sip through a straw or drinking tube to prevent staining of teeth.

Precautions:

Do not use if:
- you are receiving iron shots or injections.

Talk to your doctor if:
- you have rheumatoid arthritis, other blood diseases or anemias, colitis or other intestine problems, stomach ulcers, liver problems, or kidney problems.
- you are taking any other medication, especially acetohydroxamic acid, dimercaprol, etidronate, or tetracycline.

Side Effects:

Major:
- bluish-colored lips, fingernails, and palms of hands
- seizures
- clammy skin
- weak and fast heartbeat

Minor:
- abdominal pain, cramping, or soreness
- constipation
- dark stools
- nausea or vomiting
- darkened urine
- heartburn

Time Required for Drug to Take Effect:

Usually takes 6 months to replace iron losses.

Symptoms of Overdose:

- diarrhea
- vomiting
- bluish-colored lips, fingernails, and palms

- seizures
- drowsiness
- clammy skin
- weak and fast heart beat

Special Notes:
- Do not take iron for more than 6 months without discussing it with your doctor.
- Avoid dairy products; spinach; whole-grain breads, cereals, and bran; and tea and coffee while taking iron. These foods can decrease the amount that is absorbed. Separate the iron from these foods and drinks by at least 1 to 2 hours.
- If teeth become stained, brush with baking soda and peroxide.

fluoxetine

Brand Name: Prozac (Lilly)

Generic Available: no

Type of Drug: antidepressant (selective serotonin reuptake inhibitor)

Used for: Treatment of depression, obsessive compulsive disorder, obesity, eating disorders, and panic attacks.

How This Medication Works: Prolongs the effects of the neurotransmitter serotonin by interfering with its reuptake into nerve cells in the brain; also prolongs the actions of other neurotransmitters such as epinephrine and dopamine but to a much lesser extent.

Dosage Form and Strength:
- capsules (10 mg, 20 mg)
- liquid (20 mg/5 mL)

Storage:
- room temperature
- tightly closed

Administration:
- Usually taken once daily, usually in the morning.
- May be taken with food if medicine causes an upset stomach.

Precautions:
Do not use if:
- you have ever had an allergic reaction to fluoxetine or other selective serotonin reuptake inhibitor antidepressants such as fluvoxamine or sertraline.
- you are currently taking or have taken in the last 14 days a monoamine oxidase (MAO) inhibitor such as phenelzine or tranylcypromine.

Talk to your doctor if:
- you have ever had liver problems or kidney problems.
- you have seizures (or take medicines to control seizures), diabetes, or heart disease.
- you are taking any other type of antidepressant medicine, lithium, a cough suppressant (dextromethorphan), selegiline, warfarin, or tryptophan.

Side Effects:
Major:
- seizures
- unusual agitation or restlessness

- severe nausea or vomiting
- chest pains or palpitations
- skin rash, hives, itching
- fever and chills
- muscle or joint pain
- unusual movements of the mouth, face, arms, or legs

Minor:
- difficulty sleeping
- anxiety, nervousness
- drowsiness
- vivid dreams
- dizziness
- headache
- tremor
- blurred vision
- nausea, stomach upset
- diarrhea
- loss of appetite and weight loss
- increased appetite and weight gain
- dry mouth
- constipation
- excessive sweating
- decreased sexual function or desire

Time Required for Drug to Take Effect: May start to improve sleep or appetite within the first few weeks, but the full benefit may take from 4 to 8 weeks.

Symptoms of Overdose:
- seizures
- severe nausea and vomiting
- agitation or increased excitement

Special Notes:
- Know which "target symptoms" (restlessness, worry, fear, or changes in sleep or appetite) you are being treated for and note whether they are improving, worsening, or unchanged.
- Fluoxetine may interact with several other medicines commonly used by older adults. Show your doctor and pharmacist a complete list of all medicines, including nonprescription medicines.
- Do not drink alcohol while taking this medication.
- Never change dose without your doctor's consent.
- If you have diabetes, you may need to check your blood glucose more frequently.

flurazepam

Brand Name: Dalmane (Roche)

Generic Available: yes

Type of Drug: sedative/hypnotic

Used for: Treatment of insomnia.

How This Medication Works: Enhances the activity of the neurotransmitter gamma-aminobutyric acid.

Dosage Form and Strength: capsules (15 mg, 30 mg)

Storage:
- room temperature
- tightly closed

Administration:
- Usually taken once daily at bedtime.
- Take approximately ½ hour before you want to fall asleep.

Precautions:
Do not use if:
- you've ever had an allergic reaction to flurazepam or any other drug in the benzodiazepine family such as diazepam, lorazepam, or oxazepam.

Talk to your doctor if:
- you are taking other medications that may depress the central nervous system, including alcohol, phenobarbital, or narcotics (such as codeine, meperidine, or morphine).
- you have asthma or other lung problems, kidney disease, or liver disease.
- you have been told that you snore.
- you feel you need to continue this medicine for more than 7 days.

Side Effects:
Major:
- confusion or difficulty concentrating
- seizures
- hallucinations
- rash

Minor:
- unsteadiness
- drowsiness
- slurred speech
- blurred vision

Time Required for Drug to Take Effect: Works within 15 to 45 minutes.

Symptoms of Overdose:
- worsening confusion or slurred speech
- severe weakness or drowsiness
- shortness of breath

Special Notes:
- Flurazepam may result in a hangover effect the next day with daytime drowsiness.
- The use of flurazepam should be limited to 7 to 10 days. Longer treatment can result in REM rebound (worsening of insomnia when flurazepam is discontinued).
- Do not drink alcohol while taking this medication.
- Do not discontinue without first talking with your doctor.

fluvastatin

Brand Name: Lescol (Sandoz)

Generic Available: no

Type of Drug: antihyperlipidemic agents

Used for: Treatment of high blood cholesterol levels and cardiovascular atherosclerosis.

How This Medication Works: Decreases the amount of cholesterol manufactured in the liver by inhibiting an enzyme.

Dosage Form and Strength: tablets (20 mg, 40 mg)

Storage:
- room temperature
- tightly closed
- protected from humidity

Administration:
- Usually administered once daily.
- Take at the same time every day.
- May be taken without regard to food.

Precautions:
Do not use if:
- you are allergic to fluvastatin or similar drugs such as simvastatin, lovastatin, or pravastatin.

Talk to your doctor if:
- you have liver disease.
- you are taking any other medication, especially cyclosporine, erythromycin, warfarin, niacin, or gemfibrozil.

Side Effects:
Major:
- unexplained muscle aches
- breathing difficulty
- swelling of the face, throat, lips, or tongue

Minor:
- abdominal pain
- diarrhea
- headache
- dizziness
- taste disturbances

Time Required for Drug to Take Effect: Starts lowering blood cholesterol levels in 1 to 2 weeks, but it may take 4 to 6 weeks before reaching maximum effectiveness.

Symptoms of Overdose: No specific symptoms

Special Notes:

- Use a sunblock with at least SPF 15 when outside because fluvastatin may increase your sensitivity to the sun.
- Do not drink alcohol while taking this medication.
- Reduce your dietary cholesterol. Adhere to a low cholesterol diet.
- Fluvastatin is not a cure and must be taken on a long-term basis to have an effect.
- Your doctor will monitor your liver function with laboratory blood work while you are taking this medicine.

folic acid

Brand Name: Folvite (Lederle)

Generic Available: yes

Type of Drug: blood modifiers

Used for: Treatment of folic acid–deficiency anemia.

How This Medication Works: Replaces folic acid that is needed to make red blood cells.

Dosage Form and Strength: tablets (1 mg)

Storage:
- room temperature
- tightly closed
- protected from light

Administration:
- Usually 1 mg tablet daily.
- If you miss a dose for 1 or more days, resume your regular schedule; do not double up doses.

Precautions:
Do not take if:
- you are allergic to folic acid.
- you have pernicious anemia.

Talk to your doctor if:
- you are taking any other medications, especially methotrexate, trimethoprim, or sulfasalazine.
- you have rheumatoid arthritis, alcoholism, liver disease, other blood diseases or anemias, colitis, or intestinal problems.
- you have undergone stomach surgery or hemodialysis.

Side Effects:
Major:
- fever
- reddened skin
- shortness of breath, wheezing
- tightness in chest

Minor:
- skin rash or itching

Time Required for Drug to Take Effect:
Usually takes 1 to 2 months to replace folic acid stores.

Symptoms of Overdose:
- anorexia
- nausea
- bitter or bad taste
- depression, confusion, or altered judgement

Special Notes:
- Check with your doctor after 3 months of treatment to see how long you need to take folic acid.

furosemide

Brand Name: Lasix (Hoechst-Roussel)

Generic Available: yes

Type of Drug: diuretic

Used for: Treatment of fluid retention (edema) and high blood pressure (hypertension).

How This Medication Works: Inhibits sodium reabsorption in a specific part of the kidney, resulting in loss of water through urine.

Dosage Form and Strength:
- tablets (20 mg, 40 mg, 80 mg)
- liquid (10 mg/mL, 40 mg/5 mL)

Storage:
Tablets:
- room temperature
- tightly closed
- protected from humidity

Liquid:
- refrigerated
- tightly closed

Administration:
- Usually prescribed once or twice daily.
- Take in the morning.
- Take with food or milk if stomach upset occurs.

Precautions:
Do not use if:
- you are allergic to furosemide or the oral antidiabetic medicines such as tolazamide, glipizide, and glyburide.

Talk to your doctor if:
- you have liver disease, coronary artery disease, or gout.
- you are taking digoxin, an angiotensin-converting enzyme inhibitor (such as captopril, enalapril, or lisinopril), a thiazide diuretic (such as hydrochlorothiazide, chlorthalidone, or metolazone), warfarin, lithium, theophylline, propranolol, chloral hydrate, phenytoin, salicylates (aspirin), or nonsteroidal anti-inflammatory drugs (such as ibuprofen, diclofenac, naproxen, and oxaprozin).
- you have ever had a heart attack.
- you have diabetes or are taking an oral diabetic medication such as chlorpropamide, tolazamide, glipizide, or glyburide.

Side Effects:
Major:
- profound dehydration (thirst, rapid heart beat, weakness, fatigue, drowsiness, and dizziness)

- difficulty breathing
- muscle pain or cramps
- fainting
- chest pain
- prolonged vomiting or diarrhea

Minor:
- ringing in the ears (tinnitus)
- hearing loss
- dizziness
- dry mouth
- headache
- vertigo

Time Required for Drug to Take Effect:
Begins to work in about 45 minutes.

Symptoms of Overdose:
- acute and profound water loss
- anorexia
- lethargy
- vomiting
- mental confusion
- weakness
- dizziness

Special Notes:
- Take with orange juice or a banana to help replace lost potassium.
- Unless otherwise instructed by your doctor, it is important to drink 6 to 8 eight-ounce glasses of water daily to avoid dehydration.
- Use a sunblock with at least SPF 15 when outside because furosemide may increase your sensitivity to the sun.

- If you experience dryness of the mouth, try sugarless candy or gum, ice chips, or a saliva substitute.
- Weigh yourself daily. If you gain or lose more than 1 pound daily, call your doctor.
- Your doctor will check calcium and magnesium levels in the blood and determine if supplementation is necessary.
- Changing positions slowly when sitting and/or standing up may help decrease dizziness caused by this medication.
- If you have diabetes, you may need to check your blood glucose more frequently.

gabapentin

Brand Name: Neurontin (Parke-Davis)

Generic Available: no

Type of Drug: anticonvulsant

Used for: Prevention of seizures.

How This Medication Works: Exact mechanism is unknown.

Dosage Form and Strength: capsules (100 mg, 300 mg, 400 mg)

Storage:
- room temperature
- tightly closed
- protected from humidity

Administration:
- Usually taken 3 times daily.
- May be taken with or without meals.
- If capsules are difficult to take, they may be opened and mixed in juice or applesauce, but mix capsules immediately before you take the medication.
- If using antacids, separate doses of gabapentin and antacid by 2 hours.

Precautions:
Do not use if:
- you have had an allergic reaction to gabapentin.

Talk to your doctor if:
- you have kidney disease.
- you are taking any other medication, especially other seizure medication, antacids, cimetidine, antihistamines, sedatives, or muscle relaxants.

Side Effects:
Major:
- clumsiness
- mood changes (depression, irritability)

Minor:
- double vision
- dizziness
- drowsiness
- diarrhea
- nausea or vomiting

Time Required for Drug to Take Effect:
Therapy with this medication decreases the number and/or frequency of seizures or treats pain as long as it is continued.

Symptoms of Overdose:
- double vision
- severe diarrhea, dizziness, or drowsiness

Special Notes:
- Taking with food may reduce nausea and vomiting.
- Do not discontinue without your doctor's consent.
- Tell the doctor or dentist you are taking gabapentin if you are going to have surgery or emergency treatment.

gemfibrozil

Brand Name: Lopid (Parke-Davis)

Generic Available: yes

Type of Drug: antihyperlipidemic

Used for: Treatment of high blood cholesterol levels, high blood triglyceride levels, and cardiovascular atherosclerosis.

How This Medication Works: Decreases fatty acid uptake by the liver; inhibits the production of carrier proteins necessary for cholesterol transport.

Dosage Form and Strength:
- tablets (600 mg)
- capsules (300 mg)

Storage:
- room temperature
- tightly closed
- protected from humidity

Administration:
- Usually taken twice daily.
- Take 30 minutes before meals (breakfast and supper).

Precautions:
Do not use if:
- you are allergic to gemfibrozil or clofibrate.

Talk to your doctor if:
- you have liver disease, kidney disease, or gall-bladder disease (gallstones).
- you are taking any medication, especially warfarin or lovastatin.

Side Effects:
Major:
- unexplained muscle aches, especially if accompanied by malaise
- severe abdominal pain (gallstones)
- irregular heartbeat

Minor:
- heartburn
- feeling of fullness or bloating
- diarrhea
- fatigue
- taste alteration
- dizziness
- blurred vision

Time Required for Drug to Take Effect:
Maximum effectiveness may not be seen for 1 to 3 months.

Symptoms of Overdose: no specific symptoms

Special Notes:
- Reduce your dietary cholesterol. Adhere to a low cholesterol diet.
- Your doctor will monitor your liver function and your blood count with laboratory blood work while you are on this medicine.
- If you have diabetes, you may need to check your blood glucose more frequently.
- Do not drink alcohol while taking this medication.
- Gemfibrozil is not a cure, and you may have to take this medication for a long time.

glipizide

Brand Names:
Glucotrol (Roerig)
Glucotrol XL (Pfizer)

Generic Available:
- tablets: yes
- extended-release tablets: no

Type of Drug: hormone (antidiabetic)

Used for: Lowering glucose levels in type II (non–insulin-dependent) diabetes.

How This Medication Works: Stimulates insulin release from the pancreas and may also increase the sensitivity of the cells to insulin.

Dosage Form and Strength:
- tablets (5 mg, 10 mg)
- extended-release tablets (5 mg, 10 mg)

Storage:
- room temperature
- tightly closed
- protected from humidity

Administration:
- Usually taken once or twice daily.
- Take 30 minutes before a meal.
- Extended-release product may be taken without regard to meals.
- Take at about the same time every day.
- Do not crush or chew extended-release tablets.

Precautions:
Do not use if:
- you are allergic to glipizide or any drug in the sulfonylurea family such as glyburide, chlorpropamide, tolazamide, or tolbutamide.
- medicine is beyond the expiration date.
- you have ever had diabetic ketoacidosis.
- you have been told you have type I (insulin-dependent or juvenile-onset) diabetes.

Talk to your doctor if:
- you are taking an anticoagulant (such as warfarin), a histamine H_2 antagonist (such as ranitidine, nizatidine, famotidine, and cimetidine), a tricyclic antidepressant (such as amitriptyline, nortriptyline, desipramine, and imipramine), methyldopa, gemfibrozil, clofibrate, fenfluramine, magnesium supplements, probenecid, salicylates (aspirin), beta blockers (such as propranolol, metoprolol, atenolol, and timolol), cholestyramine, phenytoin, rifampin, thiazide diuretics

(such as hydrochlorothiazide and chlorthalidone), or digoxin.
- you have ever had liver or kidney disease.

Side Effects:

Major:
- unexplained bruising or bleeding
- hypoglycemia (sweating, shaking, headache, irritability, blurred vision, seizures, coma)
- rash or hives

Minor:
- stomach upset or fullness
- nausea
- heartburn
- diarrhea

Time Required for Drug to Take Effect:

Begins to work in 1 to 2 hours. However, you must take this medication on a regular basis to control blood glucose levels.

Symptoms of Overdose:

- profound hypoglycemia
- seizures
- coma

Special Notes:

- Do not drink alcohol while taking this medication.
- Do not discontinue without your doctor's consent.
- Talk to your doctor or diabetes educator about how to handle sick days.
- The active drug in the extended-release tablets is released through osmosis. Sometimes, the ghost of the tablet may show up in the stool and appear

not to have been absorbed. However, the active ingredient will have been absorbed.
- Use a sunblock with at least SPF 15 when outside because glipizide may increase sun sensitivity.
- When you begin glipizide therapy, check your blood glucose level frequently.

glyburide

Brand Names:

DiaBeta (Hoechst-
   Roussel)

Glynase Prestab (Upjohn)
Micronase (Upjohn)

Generic Available
- tablets: yes
- micronized tablets: no

Type of Drug: hormone (antidiabetic)

Used for: Lowering glucose levels in type II (non–insulin-dependent) diabetes.

How This Medication Works: Stimulates insulin release from the pancreas and may also increase the sensitivity of the cells to insulin.

Dosage Form and Strength:
- tablets (1.25 mg, 2.5 mg, 5 mg)
- micronized tablets (1.5 mg, 3 mg, 6 mg)

Storage:
- room temperature
- tightly closed
- protected from humidity

Administration:
- Usually taken once or twice daily.
- Take with your meals (breakfast if taking once daily; breakfast and dinner if taking twice daily).

Precautions:
Do not use if:
- you are allergic to glyburide or any drug in the sulfonylurea family such as glipizide, chlorpropamide, tolazamide, or tolbutamide.
- medicine is beyond the expiration date.
- you have ever had diabetic ketoacidosis.
- you have been told you have type I (insulin-depenent or juvenile-onset) diabetes.

Talk to your doctor if:
- you are taking an anticoagulant (such as warfarin), a histamine H_2 antagonist (such as ranitidine and cimetidine), a tricyclic antidepressant (such as amitriptyline, nortriptyline, and imipramine), methyldopa, gemfibrozil, clofibrate, fenfluramine, magnesium supplements, probenecid, salicylates (aspirin), beta blockers (such as propranolol and atenolol), cholestyramine, phenytoin, rifampin, thiazide diuretics (such as hydrochlorothiazide), or digoxin.
- you have ever had liver or kidney disease.

Side Effects:
Major:
- unexplained bruising or bleeding
- hypoglycemia (sweating, shaking, headache, irritability, blurred vision, seizures, coma)
- rash or hives

Minor:
- stomach upset or fullness
- nausea
- heartburn

Time Required for Drug to Take Effect: The nonmicronized tablets begin to work in 2 to 3 hours and continue to have an effect for about 24 hours. The micronized tablets begin to work in about 1 hour and continue to have an effect for about 24 hours.

Symptoms of Overdose:
- profound hypoglycemia
- seizures
- coma

Special Notes:
- Do not drink alcohol while taking this medication.
- Do not discontinue without first talking with your doctor.
- Talk to your doctor or diabetes educator about how to handle sick days.
- The active drug in the extended-release tablets is released through osmosis. Sometimes, the ghost of the tablet may show up in the stool, and appear not to have been absorbed. However, the active ingredient will have been absorbed.
- Use a sunblock with at least SPF 15 when outside because glyburide may increase your sensitivity to the sun.
- When you begin glyburide therapy, check your blood glucose level frequently, right before meals or 2 hours after you have eaten.

griseofulvin

Brand Names:

Gris-PEG (Allergan
  Herbert)
Fulvicin U/F, Fulvicin P/G
  (Schering)

Grifulvin V (Ortho Derm)
Grisactin Ultra (Wyeth-
  Ayerst)

Generic Available: yes

Type of Drug: antifungal

Used for: Treatment of fungal infections of the skin, hair, and nails.

How This Medication Works: Binds to keratin, a protein in skin, hair, and nails, making the tissue highly resistant to fungal invasions.

Dosage Form and Strength:

- tablets (125 mg, 165 mg, 250 mg, 330 mg, 500 mg)
- capsules (125 mg, 250 mg)
- suspension (125 mg/5 mL)

Storage:

Tablets and capsules:

- room temperature
- tightly closed
- protected from humidity

Suspension:

- room temperature
- tightly closed
- protected from light

Administration:
- Usually taken once or twice daily.
- Take at even intervals.
- Take until completely gone, even if symptoms have improved.
- Absorption will be increased by taking with a meal with a high-fat content.
- Shake suspension well before measuring dose.

Precautions:
Do not use if:
- you are allergic to griseofulvin.
- medicine is beyond the expiration date.

Talk to your doctor if:
- you are allergic to penicillin.
- you have ever had liver disease.
- you are taking warfarin, cyclosporine, phenobarbital, or aspirin.

Side Effects:
Major:
- fever, sore throat
- skin rash
- swelling of the lips or tongue
- change in the color or consistency of stools

Minor:
- nausea
- diarrhea
- dizziness

Time Required for Drug to Take Effect: Effects
may take some time, but continue to take medicine for entire course of therapy, which can be 4 to 6 months.

Symptoms of Overdose:
- nausea or vomiting
- mental confusion

Special Notes:
- Do not use for infections other than the one for which it was prescribed.
- Use a sunblock with at least SPF 15 when outside because griseofulvin may increase your sensitivity to the sun.
- Your doctor will take blood tests to monitor your blood count, kidney function, and liver function during long-term therapy.
- Treatment with a topical antifungal cream or ointment may be needed in addition to oral treatment.

haloperidol

Brand Name: Haldol (McNeil)

Generic Available: yes

Type of Drug: antipsychotic

Used for: Treatment of psychotic disorders (schizophrenia, drug-induced psychosis) and Tourette syndrome.

How This Medication Works: Blocks the neurotransmitter (dopamine) in the brain.

Dosage Form and Strength:
- tablets (0.5 mg, 1 mg, 2 mg, 5 mg, 10 mg, 20 mg)
- oral solution (2 mg/mL)

Storage:
- room temperature
- tightly closed

Administration:
- Usually taken 2 to 3 times daily.
- For the solution, dilute dose in water, orange juice, or soda; do not dilute with coffee or tea.
- Take tablets with full 8-ounce glass of water.
- Take with food or milk if stomach upset occurs.

Precautions:
Do not use if:
- you are allergic to haloperidol.

Talk to your doctor if:
- you are taking any other medications, especially antacids, phenobarbital, carbamazepine, lithium, methyldopa, phenytoin, propranolol, and tricyclic antidepressants (such as amitriptyline, imipramine).
- you have kidney or liver disease, seizures, or heart disease.

Side Effects:
Major:
- difficulty speaking or swallowing
- muscle spasms
- stiffness
- weakness

Minor:
- blurred vision
- constipation
- dry mouth
- weight gain
- nausea and vomiting

Time Required for Drug to Take Effect: May
take several days or weeks before medication's effects
are evident.

Symptoms of Overdose:
- severe dizziness
- severe drowsiness
- severe tiredness
- severe weakness
- trembling

Special Notes:
- If you experience dryness of the mouth, try sugarless candy or gum, ice, or a saliva substitute.
- Use a sunblock with at least SPF 15 when outside
  because haloperidol may increase your sensitivity
  to the sun.
- Direct contact with solution may cause a rash.

hydralazine

Brand Name: Apresoline (Ciba-Geigy)

Generic Available: yes

Type of Drug: cardiovascular (vasodilator)

Used for: Treatment of high blood pressure (hypertension), congestive heart failure, and severe aortic
insufficiency after heart valve replacement.

How This Medication Works: Acts directly on
vascular smooth muscle to cause relaxation and
widening of blood vessels.

Dosage Form and Strength: tablets (10 mg, 25 mg, 50 mg, 100 mg)

Storage:
- room temperature
- tightly closed
- protected from humidity

Administration:
- Usually taken 3 to 4 times daily; long-term therapy may be twice daily.
- Take with food.

Precautions:
Do not use if:
- you are allergic to hydralazine or tartrazine.

Talk to your doctor if:
- you have coronary artery disease, rheumatic heart disease, or obstructive lung disease.
- you have ever had a heart attack.
- you are taking propranolol, metoprolol, or indomethacin.

Side Effects:
Major:
- muscle aches, blotchy rash, fever (lupus erythematosus)
- chest pain

Minor:
- dizziness
- numbness or tingling in the arms and legs
- headache
- nausea and vomiting
- constipation

Time Required for Drug to Take Effect:
Begins to lower blood pressure in about 45 minutes.

Symptoms of Overdose:
- very rapid heartbeat
- skin flushing
- headache

Special Notes:
- Blood tests will be necessary during therapy.
- Talk to your doctor if you develop numbness or tingling in your arms or legs; pyridoxine (vitamin B_6) may alleviate these symptoms.
- Changing positions slowly when sitting and/or standing up may help decrease dizziness caused by this medication.

hydrochlorothiazide

Brand Names:
Esidrix (Ciba-Geigy)   Oretic (Abbott)
HydroDiuril (Merck)

Generic Available: yes

Type of Drug: diuretic

Used for: Treatment of fluid retention (edema) and high blood pressure (hypertension) and prevention of calcium kidney stones.

How This Medication Works: Increases the amount of sodium and chloride excretion in the kidney, resulting in loss of water through urine.

Dosage Form and Strength:
- tablets (25 mg, 50 mg, 100 mg)
- solution (50 mg/5 mL, 100 mg/mL)

Storage:
- room temperature
- tightly closed
- protected from humidity

Administration:
- Usually taken once daily, in the morning.
- Take with food or milk if stomach upset occurs.

Precautions:
Do not use if:
- you are allergic to hydrochlorothiazide or other thiazide diuretics such as chlorthalidone or metolazone.
- you are allergic to sulfa drugs such as oral diabetes medication (such as tolazamide, glipizide, or glyburide), acetazolamide, loop diuretics (such as furosemide or bumetanide), or sulfa antibacterial medication (such as sulfamethoxazole or sulfasalazine).

Talk to your doctor if:
- you have liver disease, kidney disease, or gout.
- you are taking allopurinol, warfarin, calcium supplements, digoxin, lithium, loop diuretics (such as furosemide, bumetanide, or torsemide), methyldopa, oral diabetes medication (such as tolazamide, glipizide, or glyburide), insulin, vitamin D, cholestyramine, or nonsteroidal anti-inflammatory drugs (such as ibuprofen, sulindac, indomethacin, or diclofenac).

Side Effects:

Major:
- seizures
- prolonged vomiting or diarrhea
- unexplained muscle pain, weakness, or cramps

Minor:
- headache
- dry mouth
- dizziness or drowsiness
- hyperglycemia

Time Required for Drug to Take Effect:

Begins to lower blood pressure within several days, but it may take 2 to 4 weeks for maximum effect.

Symptoms of Overdose:

- dizziness, drowsiness, lethargy, coma
- confusion
- fainting
- muscular weakness
- nausea and vomiting

Special Notes:

- Take with orange juice or a banana to help replace lost potassium.
- Unless otherwise instructed by your doctor, it is important to drink 6 to 8 eight-ounce glasses of water daily to avoid dehydration.
- Use a sunblock with at least SPF 15 when outside because hydrochlorothiazide may increase your sensitivity to the sun.
- If you experience dryness of the mouth, try sugarless candy or gum, ice chips, or a saliva substitute.

- Weigh yourself daily. If you gain or lose more than 1 pound daily, call your doctor.
- Your doctor will check calcium and magnesium levels in the blood, and determine if supplementation is necessary.
- Changing positions slowly when sitting and/or standing up may help decrease dizziness caused by this medication.
- If you have diabetes, you may need to check your blood glucose more frequently.
- You will need to have blood tests done periodically during therapy.
- The diuretic effect of hydrochlorothiazide may become less noticeable with continued therapy, but it continues to exert a blood pressure–lowering effect.

hydrocodone and acetaminophen combination

Brand Names:

Amacodone (Trimen)
Anexsia (ECR Pharm)
Bancap HC (Forest)
Co-Gesic (Central)
Dolacet (Hauck)
Duradyne DHC (Forest)

Hydrogesic (Edwards)
Hy-Phen (Ascher)
Lorcet (UAD)
Lortab (Whitby)
Vicodin (Knoll)
Vicodin ES (Knoll)

Generic Available: yes

Type of Drug: analgesic

Used for: Relief of pain.

How This Medication Works: Hydrocodone acts in the central nervous system to decrease the recognition of pain impulses. Acetaminophen works in the peripheral nervous system and blocks pain impulses.

Dosage Form and Strength:
- tablets (2.5 mg/500 mg, 5 mg/500 mg, 7.5 mg/ 500 mg, 7.5 mg/650 mg, 7.5 mg/750 mg)
- capsules (5 mg/500 mg)
- liquid (2.5 mg/167 mg per 5 mL)

Storage:
- room temperature
- protected from humidity

Administration:
- Do not exceed the maximum number of doses per day. Each agent can be harmful if used in excess. Never take more tablets per dose, or doses per day than your doctor has prescribed.
- Take with food or milk if stomach upset occurs.

Precautions:
Do not use if:
- you are allergic to hydrocodone or other narcotics such as morphine, codeine, hydromorphone, or oxycodone.
- you are allergic to acetaminophen.

Talk to your doctor if:
- you have alcoholism or other substance abuse problems; brain disease or head injury; colitis; seizures; emotional problems or mental illness; emphysema, asthma, or other lung diseases;

kidney, liver, or thyroid disease; prostate problems or problems with urination or gallbladder disease or gallstones.
- you are taking naltrexone, zidovudine, or any other medications, especially those that can cause drowsiness such as antihistamines, barbiturates (phenobarbital), benzodiazepines (diazepam, alprazolam, lorazepam), muscle relaxants, or antidepressants.

Side Effects:
Major:
- skin rash or hives
- difficulty breathing
- fainting
- fast, slow, or pounding heartbeat
- frequent urge to urinate
- painful or difficult urination
- hallucinations
- depression
- pinpoint red spots on body
- unusual bruising or bleeding
- trembling or uncontrolled muscle movements
- yellow eyes or skin (jaundice)

Minor:
- nausea
- constipation
- drowsiness
- dry mouth
- general feeling of discomfort or illness
- loss of appetite
- difficulty sleeping
- nervousness or restlessness

Time Required for Drug to Take Effect: Starts to work within 15 to 30 minutes.

Symptoms of Overdose:
- cold, clammy skin
- severe confusion
- seizures
- severe dizziness or drowsiness
- protracted nausea, vomiting, or diarrhea
- severe nervousness or restlessness
- shortness of breath or difficulty breathing
- slowed heartbeat

(Symptoms associated with acetaminophen may not occur until 2 to 4 days after the overdose is taken, but it is important to begin treatment as soon as possible after the overdose to prevent liver damage or death.)

Special Notes:
- This medication may cause drowsiness. Do not operate a motor vehicle or other machinery while you are taking this medication.
- Hydrocodone, morphine, and other narcotics (oxycodone, codeine) cause constipation. This side effect may be diminished by drinking 6 to 8 full glasses of water each day. If using this medication for chronic pain, adding a stool softener–laxative combination may be necessary.
- Check with your physician or pharmacist before using any over-the-counter medications.
- When hydrocodone is used over a long period of time, your body may become tolerant and require larger doses.

- Do not stop taking this medication abruptly or you may experience symptoms of withdrawal.
- Nausea and vomiting may occur, especially after the first few doses. This effect may go away if you lie down for a while.
- If you experience dry mouth, try sugarless candy or gum, ice chips, or a saliva substitute.
- Do not drink alcohol while taking this medication.

hydroxychloroquine

Brand Name: Plaquenil (Sanofi Winthrop)

Generic Available: no

Type of Drug: antirheumatic

Used for: Treatment of rheumatoid arthritis (to slow the disease progress).

How This Medicine Works: Prevents the formation of substances in the body responsible for the inflammation that causes rheumatoid arthritis; may also block the action of certain enzymes that destroy collagen tissues in the joints.

Dosage Form and Strength: tablets (200 mg)

Storage:
- room temperature
- tightly closed

Administration:
- Usually 1 to 3 daily.
- Take with food or milk if stomach upset occurs.

Precautions:

Do not use if:
- you are allergic to hydroxychloroquine.
- you have experienced eye damage as a result of using hydroxychloroquine.
- you have ever had a problem with psoriasis or been told you have porphyria.

Talk to your doctor if:
- you have ever had any problems with your liver.
- you have anemia or other blood disorders.
- you are taking digoxin or medicine for stomach problems.

Side Effects:

Major:
- vision changes
- severe headache
- severe nausea or vomiting
- severe muscle weakness
- seizures
- difficulty breathing
- fainting
- nightmares
- severe agitation or confusion
- ringing in the ears (tinnitus)
- fever or sore throat
- unusual bleeding, easy bruising

Minor:
- stomach upset
- drowsiness

Time Required for Drug to Take Effect: May take months to see the full benefit of treatment.

Symptoms of Overdose:
- severe headache
- severe drowsiness
- seizures
- change in vision
- fainting
- nausea and vomiting

Special Notes:
- Regular visits to the eye doctor are required when using this medicine.
- This medicine has also been used for several other conditions such as the prevention of malaria and the treatment of certain types of skin problems.
- You may need to have blood tests done periodically during therapy.

hydroxyzine

Brand Names:
Atarax (Roerig)
Vistaril (Pfizer)

Generic Available: yes

Type of Drug: antihistamine

Used for: Treatment of anxiety and itching.

How This Medication Works: Blocks histamine—a substance that causes sneezing, itching, and runny nose; can also cause drowsiness as a side effect, which is used when prescribed for anxiety.

Dosage Form and Strength:
- tablets (10 mg, 25 mg, 50 mg, 100 mg)
- capsules (25 mg, 50 mg, 100 mg)
- suspension (25 mg/5 mL)
- syrup (10 mg/5 mL)

Storage:
- room temperature
- protected from humidity

Administration:
- Shake the suspension well before measuring out the appropriate dose.
- Use a measuring device that can measure in milliliters (mL or ml); an ordinary teaspoon is not accurate enough.
- Take with food or milk if stomach upset occurs.

Precautions:
Do not use if:
- you are allergic to hydroxyzine or other antihistamines such as diphenhydramine, terfenadine, or cyproheptadine.

Talk to your doctor if:
- you have asthma, enlarged prostate, difficulty urinating, or glaucoma.
- you are taking any other medications, especially antidepressants or antibiotics.

Side Effects:
Major:
- skin rash, hives, or itching
- sore throat or fever
- hallucinations

- feeling faint
- seizures or convulsions
- difficulty breathing
- nervousness or restlessness

Minor:
- drowsiness, dizziness, or confusion
- thickening of mucous
- blurred vision
- difficult or painful urination
- irregular heartbeat
- increased sensitivity to sun
- increased sweating
- increased appetite
- nightmares

Time Required for Drug to Take Effect: Starts to work within 15 to 30 minutes.

Symptoms of Overdose:
- dry mouth, throat, or nose
- flushed skin
- dilated pupils
- difficulty breathing
- dizziness or drowsiness
- excitation

Special Notes:
- Tell the doctor you are taking hydroxyzine before you have skin tests for allergies.
- Do not drink alcohol or take other medications that cause drowsiness or mental slowing.
- This medication may cause drowsiness. Do not operate a motor vehicle or other machinery while you are taking this medication.

- If you experience dryness of the mouth, try sugarless candy or gum, ice chips, or a saliva substitute.
- Tell the doctor or dentist you are taking hydroxyzine if you are going to have surgery or emergency treatment.

ibuprofen

Brand Names:

Motrin (Upjohn)
Advil (Whitehall-Robins)
Haltran (Roberts)
Nuprin (Bristol-Myers)

Ibuprofen Oral Suspension (UDL, Xactdose)

Generic Available: yes

Type of Drug: nonsteroidal anti-inflammatory drug (analgesic, anti-inflammatory, and antipyretic)

Used for: Treatment of pain associated with rheumatoid arthritis, osteoarthritis, headache, toothache, dental procedures, muscular aches, orthopedic procedures, backache, athletic injuries, and miscellaneous aches and pains; can also be used to reduce a fever.

How This Medication Works: Inhibits substances called prostaglandins that cause pain and inflammation.

Dosage Form and Strength:

- tablets (100 mg, 200 mg, 300 mg, 400 mg, 600 mg, 800 mg)
- tablets, chewable (50 mg, 100 mg)
- liquid/oral suspension (100 mg/5 mL)

Storage:
- room temperature
- tightly closed
- protected from moisture and light

Administration:
- Usually taken 3 or 4 times daily.
- For nonprescription, you may take 200 to 400 mg every 4 to 6 hours, up to 1200 mg per 24 hours.
- Take with meals or milk if stomach upset occurs.
- Take with a full glass of water (6 to 8 ounces).
- Shake suspension well before measuring dose.

Precautions:
Do not use if:
- you are allergic to ibuprofen or any other non-steroidal anti-inflammatory drug such as etodolac, indomethacin, piroxicam, or aspirin.
- medicine is beyond the expiration date or looks unusual.

Talk to your doctor if:
- you are taking aspirin; another nonsteroidal anti-inflammatory drug such as etodolac, indometh-acin, or piroxicam; anticoagulants such as warfarin; steroids such as prednisone; or lithium.
- you have peptic ulcer disease, bleeding from your stomach or intestines, bleeding abnormalities, high blood pressure (hypertension), kidney disease, liver disease, or heart disease.

Side Effects:
Major:
- blood in stool or dark, tarry stool
- persistent or severe stomach or abdominal pain

- vomiting blood
- blood in urine or dark, smokey-colored urine
- difficulty urinating
- rash
- difficulty breathing
- swelling of the eyelids, throat, lips, or face (allergic reaction)
- vision or hearing changes

Minor:
- stomach upset
- swelling of hands or feet
- dizziness
- drowsiness

Time Required for Drug to Take Effect: Starts
to relieve pain in 1 to 2 hours. However, it may take
1 to 2 weeks to feel the full benefits of this medicine
when treating arthritis.

Symptoms of Overdose:
- stomach pain
- nausea and vomiting
- drowsiness
- headache
- ringing in the ears (tinnus)
- seizures
- irregular heartbeat

Special Notes:
- Some chewable tablets contain aspartame, which
  may be a concern if you have a history of
  phenylketonuria, or if you have been told to limit
  your intake of phenylalanine.

- Alcohol may increase your risk of bleeding from the stomach or intestines while taking ibuprofen.
- Contact your physician if pain or fever worsens during self-treatment.
- Self-medication with ibuprofen should not exceed 10 days unless otherwise directed by a physician or pharmacist. Self-medication of fever should not exceed 3 days unless otherwise directed by a physician or pharmacist.

imipramine

Brand Names:
Janimine (Abbott)   Tofranil-PM (Ciba-Geigy)
Tofranil (Ciba-Geigy)

Generic Available: yes

Type of Drug: tricyclic antidepressant

Used for: Treatment of depression, chronic pain, and urinary incontinence.

How This Medication Works: Increases the action of the neurotransmitters norepinephrine and serotonin in the brain.

Dosage Form and Strength:
- tablets (10 mg, 25 mg, 50 mg)
- capsules (75 mg, 100 mg, 125 mg, 150 mg)

Storage:
- room temperature
- tightly closed

Administration:
- Usually taken once daily at bedtime; may also be prescribed 2 to 3 times daily.
- Capsules are only prescribed at bedtime.
- May be taken without regard to food.

Precautions:
Do not use if:
- you have had an allergic reaction to imipramine or any other tricyclic antidepressant such as amitriptyline or desipramine.
- you are also taking (or have taken in the past 14 days) a monoamine oxidase (MAO) inhibitor such as phenelzine or selegiline.

Talk to your doctor if:
- you have glaucoma (angle closure type), heart disease, urinary or prostate problems, severe constipation, breathing problems, seizures, diabetes, or a thyroid problem.
- you are taking cimetidine, clonidine, methyldopa, reserpine, guanethidine, sedatives, muscle relaxants, antihistamines, decongestants (including cold medications), or stimulants.
- you drink alcohol on a regular or occasional basis.

Side Effects:
Major:
- dizziness with falls
- fainting
- rapid heartbeat
- chest pain
- confusion

- severe constipation
- urinary retention
- rash
- severe sedation
- fever
- hallucinations
- restlessness
- agitation
- severe sunburn

Minor:
- drowsiness
- dry mouth
- mild constipation
- weight gain
- unpleasant taste
- stomach upset

Time Required for Drug to Take Effect: May take from 4 to 8 weeks for full antidepressant benefit; improvement may occur within 1 to 2 weeks for certain types of pain.

Symptoms of Overdose:
- confusion
- hallucinations
- seizures
- extreme sedation
- very slow or rapid heartbeat
- low blood pressure
- difficulty breathing
- inability to urinate
- severe constipation
- dilated pupils

Special Notes:

- Know which "target symptoms" (restlessness, worry, fear, or changes in sleep or appetite) you are being treated for and be prepared to tell your doctor if your target symptoms are improving, worsening, or unchanged.
- Your doctor may order a blood test to determine the level of imipramine in your body.
- If you are taking this medicine for urinary incontinence, your doctor may suggest that you keep a record of incontinence episodes.
- Do not discontinue without your doctor's consent.
- Never increase your dose without the advice of your doctor.
- Check with your physician or pharmacist before using any over-the-counter medications.
- If you have diabetes, you may need to check your blood glucose more frequently.
- Use a sunblock with at least SPF 15 when outside because imipramine may increase your sensitivity to the sun.

indomethacin

Brand Names:
Indocin (Merck)
Indocin CR (Merck)

Generic Available: yes

Type of Drug: nonsteroidal anti-inflammatory drug
(analgesic, anti-inflammatory, and antipyretic)

Used for: Relief of pain associated with rheumatoid arthritis, osteoarthritis, gouty arthritis, ankylosing spondylitis, surgery recovery, headache, and bursitis; can also be used to reduce a fever.

How This Medication Works: Inhibits substances called prostaglandins that cause pain and inflammation.

Dosage Form and Strength:
- capsule (25 mg, 50 mg)
- extended-release capsule (75 mg)
- oral suspension (25 mg/5 mL)
- rectal suppository (50 mg)

Storage:
Liquid/oral suspension, capsules and extended-release capsules:
- room temperature
- tightly closed
- protected from moisture and light

Rectal suppositories:
- store as directed (sometimes refrigerated)

Administration:
Capsules or suspension:
- Usually taken 2 or 3 times daily.
- Take with meals or milk to minimize stomach upset.
- Do not lie down for at least 30 minutes after taking this medicine.
- Take with a full glass of water (6 to 8 ounces).
- Do not break, crush, or chew extended-release tablets.

- Shake suspension well before measuring dose.
- Moisten the suppository before insertion.
- If suppository is too soft at the time of administration, chill in the refrigerator for 30 minutes or run cold water over it before removing the wrapper.
- Suppository must be retained in the rectum for at least 1 hour to maximize absorption.

Precautions:

Do not use if:

- you are allergic to indomethacin or any other nonsteroidal anti-inflammatory drug such as etodolac, ibuprofen, piroxicam, or aspirin.
- medicine is beyond the expiration date or looks unusual in appearance.

Talk to your doctor if:

- you are taking aspirin; another nonsteroidal anti-inflammatory drug such as ibuprofen, etodolac, or piroxicam; anticoagulants such as warfarin; steroids such as prednisone; lithium; beta blockers such as atenolol; diuretics such as furosemide or hydrochlorothiazide; diabetes medication; or methotrexate.
- you have peptic ulcer disease, bleeding from your stomach or intestines, bleeding abnormalities, ulcerative colitis, high blood pressure (hypertension), kidney disease, liver disease, heart disease, asthma, or nasal polyps.
- you smoke tobacco or drink alcohol.
- your doctor has ordered rectal indomethacin suppositories and you have a history of hemorrhoids, prostate problems, or anal or rectal inflammation or bleeding.

Side Effects:

Major:
- blood in stool or dark, tarry stool
- persistent or severe stomach or abdominal pain
- vomiting blood
- blood in urine or dark, smokey-colored urine
- difficulty urinating
- rash
- difficulty breathing
- swelling of the eyelids, throat, lips, or face
- vision or hearing changes
- unexplained sore throat or fever
- unusual bleeding or bruising

Minor:
- stomach upset, gas, or heartburn
- diarrhea or constipation
- swelling of hands or feet
- dizziness
- drowsiness
- headache

Time Required for Drug to Take Effect: Starts
to relieve pain in 1 to 2 hours. However, it may take
1 to 2 weeks to feel the full benefits of this medicine
when treating arthritis.

Symptoms of Overdose:
- stomach pain
- nausea and vomiting
- drowsiness
- headache
- seizures
- heartburn

Special Notes:
- Drinking alcohol or smoking tobacco may increase your risk of bleeding from the stomach or intestines.
- Indomethacin contains sodium, which may worsen heart failure, high blood pressure (hypertension), and ankle edema.
- Tell the doctor or dentist you are taking indomethacin if you are going to have surgery or emergency treatment.
- Contact physician if pain or fever worsens during treatment.

insulin

Brand Names:
Iletin (Lilly)   Novolin (Novo Nordisk)
Humulin (Lilly)

Generic Available: no

Type of Drug: hormone (antidiabetic)

Used for: Lowering glucose levels in type I (insulin-dependent or juvenile-onset) diabetes and type II (non–insulin-dependent or adult-onset) diabetes.

How This Medication Works: Allows glucose to enter cells from the bloodstream.

Dosage Form and Strength: There are several different sources, types, and concentrations of insulin available; all are injections. (See "Time Required for Drug to Take Effect" and "Special Notes" below.)

Storage:
- refrigerated (Room temperature is OK for up to 28 days; never freeze or use insulin that has been frozen.)
- protected from light

Administration:
- Take your insulin at about the same times every day (relative to meals).
- Roll the bottle gently between your palms to mix long-acting insulin (NPH, lente, ultralente). Never shake your insulin hard.
- Inject into the same general area (for example, the abdomen), but change the exact site of the injection with each dose.
- Injection in the abdomen will give the most predictable rate of absorption; injection into the fleshy portion of the upper arms or into the legs will be affected by exercise of the extremities.
- Some people can control their diabetes with 1 injection daily, but most people require 2 or more shots every day.
- Regular insulin should be taken 45 to 60 minutes before a meal. The rate of absorption depends on the size of the dose; the larger the dose, the slower the rate of absorption.

Precautions:
Do not use if:
- you have had a previous allergic reaction to the same species of insulin. (Because of the sources and the way they are produced, it is possible to be allergic to one kind of insulin and not to another.)

- medicine is beyond the expiration date.
- medicine has an unusual appearance—cloudy, thickened, slightly colored, or has any solid particles in it for regular insulin; stays at the bottom of the bottle after gentle shaking or has clumps or solid particles that stick to the bottom or sides of the bottle after gentle shaking (is "frosted") for semilente, NPH, lente, ultralente, 70/30, or 50/50.

Talk to your doctor if:
- you are taking a loop or thiazide diuretic such as furosemide or hydrochlorothiazide.

Side Effects:
Major:
- very low blood sugar (sweating, shaking, headache, irritability, blurred vision, seizures, coma)
- difficulty breathing
- rash or hives
- unexplained muscle aches or cramps

Minor:
- irritation at site of injection

Time Required for Drug to Take Effect: There are several types of insulin, each with a different onset and duration of action. The times given below are estimates; each insulin may work a little differently in your body.

- Regular insulin and semilente are short-acting insulin. They have peak effect in about 1 hour and will last for 6 to 8 hours.
- NPH and lente insulin are intermediate-acting insulin. They reach peak effect in about 6 to 8 hours and will last 18 to 24 hours.

- Mixtures of regular and NPH (either 70/30 or 50/50) combine the actions of the two types. For example, in an injection of 70/30, 30% of the dose peaks in 1 hour and lasts for 6 to 8 hours (regular), and 70% of the dose peaks in 6 to 8 hours and last for 18 to 24 hours (NPH).
- Ultralente is a long-acting insulin. It reaches peak effect in 6 to 16 hours and lasts 27 to 29 hours.

Symptoms of Overdose:
- profound hypoglycemia
- seizures
- coma

Special Notes:
- Dietary management and regular physical activity remain important methods of controlling blood glucose levels.
- Do not discontinue without first talking with your doctor.
- Talk to your doctor or diabetes educator about how to handle sick days.
- Do not drink alcohol while taking this medication.
- When you begin insulin therapy, check your blood glucose level frequently, right before meals or 2 hours after you have eaten.
- Absorption of insulin depends on the size of the dose and the site of the injection.
- Make sure that you get exactly the kind that your doctor wants you to have. Using the wrong insulin can seriously affect your glucose control.
- You must know the species of your insulin: human, pork, or a mixture of beef and pork.

- You must know the brand name of your insulin.
- You must know the type of insulin that you take. There is a large letter or number on the insulin bottle that shows the type of insulin: regular insulin (R), semilente insulin (S), NPH insulin (N), lente insulin (L), ultralente (U), 70% NPH and 30% regular (70/30), or 50% NPH and 50% regular (50/50).
- You must know the concentration of your insulin (100 units per cc is the most commonly used; 500 units per cc is available by prescription).
- The syringes that you buy must match the concentration of your insulin.

insulin lispro

Brand Name: Humalog (Lilly)

Generic Available: no

Type of Drug: hormone (antidiabetic)

Used for: Lowering glucose levels in type I (insulin-dependent or juvenile-onset) diabetes and type II (non–insulin-dependent or adult-onset) diabetes.

How This Medication Works: Allows glucose to enter cells from the bloodstream.

Dosage Form and Strength:
- injection vial (100 units/cc)
- cartridges (1.5 cc) for use with insulin "pen"

(One unit of insulin lispro is equivalent to 1 unit of regular insulin.)

Storage:
- refrigerated (Room temperature is OK for up to 28 days; never freeze or use insulin that has been frozen.)
- protected from light

Administration:
- Insulin lispro is injected subcutaneously (under the skin) 15 minutes before a meal.
- Insulin lispro can be used in twice-daily or multiple daily injections.
- Insulin lispro's fast absorption means patients can tailor their insulin dosing to meals rather than plan meals based on their insulin dosing.

Precautions:
Do not use if:
- you have had an allergic reaction to insulin or insulin lispro.
- medicine is beyond the expiration date.

Talk to your doctor if:
- you are taking a loop or thiazide diuretic such as furosemide or hydrochlorothiazide.

Side Effects:
Major:
- very low blood sugar (sweating, shaking, headache, irritability, nervousness, blurred vision, seizures, coma)
- difficulty breathing
- rash or hives
- unexplained muscle aches or cramps

Minor:
- irritation at site of injection

Time Required for Drug to Take Effect:

Begins to work after 15 minutes and reaches its peak action in 30 to 90 minutes, coinciding with the body's need for insulin after a meal. Insulin lispro's duration of action is about 4 or 5 hours.

Symptoms of Overdose:

- profound hypoglycemia
- seizures
- coma

Special Notes:

- Dietary management and regular physical activity remain important methods of controlling blood glucose levels.
- Do not discontinue without first talking with your doctor.
- Talk to your doctor or diabetes educator about how to handle sick days.
- Do not drink alcohol while taking this medication.
- When you begin insulin therapy, check your blood glucose level frequently, right before meals or 2 hours after you have eaten.
- Unlike other insulin, insulin lispro requires a doctor's prescription.
- Due to its short duration of action, patients with type I (insulin-dependent or juvenile-onset) diabetes will also require a long-acting insulin such as NPH or ultralente.
- Insulin lispro can be mixed in the same syringe with NPH, lente, or ultralente insulin. These mixtures should be injected immediately after mixing.

ipratropium

Brand Name: Atrovent (Boehringer Ingelheim)

Generic Available: no

Type of Drug: respiratory (antiasthma, antiallergic)

Used for: Treatment of emphysema and chronic bronchitis.

How This Medication Works: Causes the passageways in the lungs to dilate.

Dosage Form and Strength: inhaler (18 µg/inhalation)

Storage:
- room temperature
- protected from humidity

Administration:
- Have your doctor or pharmacist demonstrate the proper procedure for using the inhaler and make sure you practice your technique in front of them.
- Allow at least 2 minutes between inhalations (puffs).
- If you have more than one inhaler, it is important to administer your inhalers in the correct order. If you are using albuterol and ipratropium, use the albuterol first. Wait at least 5 minutes before inhaling the ipratropium. If you are using albuterol, ipratropium, and a steroid inhaler, use the albuterol first, then the ipratropium, then the steroid inhaler.

Precautions:

Do not use if:
- you are allergic to ipratropium or other anti-cholinergic drugs such as atropine, belladonna, hyoscyamine, or scopolamine.

Talk to your doctor if:
- you have difficulty urinating or enlarged prostate.
- you are taking any other medications.

Side Effects:

Major:
- skin rash, hives, or itching
- ulcers or sores in the mouth or on the lips
- blurred vision
- difficulty urinating
- irregular heartbeat

Minor:
- cough or dryness of mouth or throat
- headache or dizziness
- nervousness
- stomach upset or nausea
- metallic or unpleasant taste
- stuffy nose
- trembling
- difficulty sleeping

Time Required for Drug to Take Effect: Starts to work within 1 to 3 minutes.

Symptoms of Overdose:
- blurred vision
- headache
- nervousness
- dry mouth or drying of respiratory secretions

- cough
- nausea

Special Notes:
- Check with your physician and pharmacist before you use any over-the-counter medications.
- Be sure that you keep track of how many inhalations are left and get your medication refilled about 1 week before you expect to run out.
- Sometimes a spacer device is used with your inhaler. This device helps the medication get to the lungs instead of the mouth or throat.

isoniazid

Brand Name: Laniazid (Lannett)

Generic Available: yes

Type of Drug: antitubercular

Used for: Prevention of infection in persons exposed to tuberculosis and treatment of active tuberculosis.

How This Medication Works: Inhibits the growth of the organism that causes tuberculosis.

Dosage Form and Strength:
- tablets (50 mg, 100 mg, 300 mg)
- syrup (50 mg/5 mL)

Storage:
- room temperature
- tightly closed
- protected from humidity

Administration:

- Generally taken once daily.
- Take at about the same time every day.
- For best absorption, take on an empty stomach; however, it may be taken with food if stomach upset occurs.
- If using antacids, separate doses of isoniazid and antacid by 2 hours.

Precautions:

Do not use if:
- you are allergic to isoniazid.
- medicine is beyond the expiration date.

Talk to your doctor if:
- you have liver disease.
- you are taking warfarin, carbamazepine, phenytoin, disulfiram, ketoconazole, meperidine, rifampin, or any drug in the benzodiazepine family such as diazepam or temazepam.

Side Effects:

Major:
- yellowing of the skin or eyes (jaundice)
- dark urine and/or pale stools
- numbness or tingling in the hands or feet

Minor:
- nausea
- stomach upset

Time Required for Drug to Take Effect:

Begins to kill infecting organisms within hours after taking your first dose. However, you must continue to take isoniazid for the full course of treatment, even if symptoms disappear.

Symptoms of Overdose:
- vomiting
- dizziness or slurred speech
- hallucinations
- shortness of breath
- coma

Special Notes:
- Minimize your alcohol intake while on isoniazid. Use of alcohol will increase the risk of liver damage.
- Supplementation with vitamin B_6 may be necessary while you are on isoniazid.
- Foods rich in histamine such as tuna, sauerkraut juice, and yeast extract may cause headache, sweating, flushing, diarrhea, or itching.
- Aged foods rich in tyramine such as salami, red wines, pepperoni, Brie, Camembert, cheddar cheese, and fava beans may cause dangerously high blood pressure.

isosorbide dinitrate

Brand Names:
Isordil (Wyeth-Ayerst)   Dilatrate-SR (Reedco)
Sorbitrate (Zeneca)

Generic Available: yes

Type of Drug: antianginal

Used for: Treatment of congestive heart failure, angina, and coronary heart disease.

How This Medication Works: Relaxes smooth muscle, reducing blood pressure and demand on the heart.

Dosage Form and Strength:
- tablets (5 mg, 10 mg, 20 mg, 30 mg, 40 mg)
- sublingual tablets (2.5 mg, 5 mg, 10 mg)
- chewable tablets (5 mg, 10 mg)
- sustained-release tablets and capsules (40 mg)

Storage:
- room temperature
- tightly closed in original container
- protected from humidity

Administration:
- Oral or sustained-release products are usually taken 3 or 4 times daily.
- Sublingual and chewable tablets are taken when necessary to relieve chest pain.
- It is important to have an 8- to 10-hour period each day that is drug-free. If the drug is taken continuously, tolerance will develop and the medication will become ineffective. If dosing 4 times daily, take the tablets at 9 A.M., 1 P.M., 5 P.M., and 9 P.M.
- Take on an empty stomach, 1 hour before or 2 hours after a meal.
- Take tablets with a full glass of water.
- Dissolve sublingual tablets slowly under the tongue; do not swallow, crush, or chew.
- Use sublingual tablets when seated.
- Swallow sustained-release tablets or capsules; do not crush or chew.

Precautions:

Do not use if:
- you are allergic to isosorbide dinitrate or other medicines in the nitrate family such as nitro-glycerin and isosorbide mononitrate.
- medicine is beyond the expiration date.

Talk to your doctor if:
- you have glaucoma or severe anemia.
- you are taking a calcium channel blocker such as nifedipine, diltiazem, verapamil, or felodipine.

Side Effects:

Major:
- fainting
- chest pain
- blurred vision
- dry mouth

Minor:
- headache
- nausea and diarrhea
- weakness
- flushing

Time Required for Drug to Take Effect:

Sublingual tablets begin to work in 2 to 5 minutes; oral tablets begin to work in about 30 minutes and continue to have an effect for 4 to 6 hours; sustained-release tablets and capsules begin to work in about 4 hours and continue to work for up to 8 hours.

Symptoms of Overdose:

- rapid heartbeat
- visual disturbances
- shortness of breath

Special Notes:

- Changing positions slowly when sitting and/or standing up may help decrease dizziness caused by this medication.
- If you notice dizziness, avoid activities requiring mental alertness, such as operating a motor vehicle or operating dangerous machinery.
- Do not drink alcohol while taking this medication.
- Do not change from one brand of this drug to another without consulting your pharmacist or physician.
- Use sublingual or chewable tablets for acute angina attacks.
- Do not use nonchewable tablets for acute angina attacks.
- The active drug in the extended-release tablets is released through osmosis. Sometimes, the ghost of the tablet may show up in the stool, and appear not to have been absorbed. However, the active ingredient will have been absorbed.

isosorbide mononitrate

Brand Names:

Monoket (Schwarz
  Pharma)

ISMO (Wyeth-Ayerst)
Imdur (Key)

Generic Available: no

Type of Drug: antianginal

Used for: Treatment of congestive heart failure, angina, and coronary heart disease.

How This Medication Works: Relaxes smooth muscle, reducing blood pressure and demand on the heart.

Dosage Form and Strength: tablets (10 mg, 20 mg, 40 mg)

Storage:
- room temperature
- tightly closed in original container
- protected from humidity

Administration:
- Usually taken once or twice daily.
- It is important to have an 8- to 10-hour period each day that is drug-free. If taken continuously, tolerance will develop and the medication becomes ineffective. If dosing twice daily, take tablets 7 hours apart (9 A.M. and 4 P.M.).
- Take on an empty stomach, 1 hour before or 2 hours after meals.
- Take with a glassful of water.

Precautions:
Do not use if:
- you are allergic to isosorbide mononitrate or other medicines in the nitrate family such as nitroglycerin and isosorbide dinitrate.
- medicine is beyond the expiration date.

Talk to your doctor if:
- you have glaucoma or severe anemia.
- you are taking a calcium channel blocker such as nifedipine, amlodipine, diltiazem, verapamil, or felodipine.

Side Effects:

Major:
- fainting
- chest pain
- blurred vision
- dry mouth

Minor:
- headache
- nausea
- weakness
- diarrhea
- stomach upset
- flushing

Time Required for Drug to Take Effect:

Begins to have effect in about 1 hour.

Symptoms of Overdose:

- very low blood pressure
- rapid heartbeat
- visual disturbances
- shortness of breath

Special Notes:

- Changing positions slowly when sitting and/or standing up may help decrease dizziness caused by this medication.
- If you notice dizziness, avoid activities requiring mental alertness, such as operating a motor vehicle or operating dangerous machinery.
- Do not drink alcohol while taking this medication.
- Do not use tablets for acute angina attacks.

itraconazole

Brand Name: Sporanox (Janssen)

Generic Available: no

Type of Drug: antifungal

Used for: Treatment of fungal infections.

How This Medication Works: Interrupts the formation of fungal cell membranes.

Dosage Form and Strength: capsules (100 mg)

Storage:
- room temperature
- tightly closed
- protected from humidity

Administration:
- Usually taken once daily.
- Take with food to increase absorption.

Precautions:
Do not use if:
- you are allergic to itraconazole or any of the -azole antifungal family such as ketoconazole.
- medicine is beyond the expiration date.

Talk to your doctor if:
- you are taking terfenadine, astemizole, cyclosporine, digoxin, warfarin, isoniazid, phenytoin, rifampin, oral diabetes medication (such as glyburide, glipizide, or tolazamide), or a histamine H_2 antagonist (such as cimetidine or ranitidine).
- you have ever had liver disease.

Side Effects:

Major:
- persistent vomiting or diarrhea
- fever and malaise
- rash
- unexplained muscle aches or cramps
- yellowing of the skin or eyes (jaundice)
- dark urine and/or pale stools

Minor:
- nausea
- abdominal pain
- headache
- dizziness

Time Required for Drug to Take Effect: Effects

may not be seen for some time, but continue to take this medicine for the entire course of therapy, which can be anywhere from 1 day to 6 months.

Symptoms of Overdose:
- hallucinations
- urinary incontinence
- seizures

Special Notes:
- Do not use for infections other than the one for which it was prescribed.

ketoconazole

Brand Name: Nizoral (Janssen)

Generic Available: no

Type of Drug: antifungal

Used for: Treatment of fungal infections of the skin, hair, and nails.

How This Medication Works: Interrupts the formation of fungal cell membranes.

Dosage Form and Strength: tablets (200 mg)

Storage:
- room temperature
- tightly closed
- protected from humidity

Administration:
- Take at about the same time every day.
- Take on an empty stomach, at least 1 hour before or 2 hours after a meal.
- May be taken with food if stomach upset occurs.
- If using antacids, separate doses of ketoconazole and antacid by 2 hours.

Precautions:
Do not use if:
- you are allergic to ketoconazole or any other -azole antifungal such as itraconazole.
- medicine is beyond the expiration date.

Talk to your doctor if:
- you are taking terfenadine, astemizole, cyclosporine, warfarin, isoniazid, phenytoin, rifampin, theophylline, prednisone, oral diabetes medication (such as glyburide or glipizide), or a histamine H_2 antagonist (such as cimetidine or ranitidine).
- you have ever had liver disease.

Side Effects:

Major:
- persistent vomiting or diarrhea
- fever and malaise
- rash
- unexplained muscle aches or cramps
- yellowing of the skin or eyes (jaundice)
- dark urine and/or pale stools

Minor:
- nausea
- abdominal pain
- headache
- dizziness
- drowsiness

Time Required for Drug to Take Effect: Effects
may not be seen for some time, but continue to take this medicine for the entire course of therapy, which can be anywhere from 1 day to 6 months.

Symptoms of Overdose:
- hallucinations
- urinary incontinence
- seizures

Special Notes:
- Do not use for infections other than the one for which it was prescribed.
- This medication may cause drowsiness. Use caution when operating a motor vehicle or operating dangerous machinery.
- The doctor will take blood tests to monitor your liver function if you take ketoconazole for more than a few weeks.

ketorolac

Brand Name: Toradol (Syntex)

Generic Available: no

Type of Drug: nonsteroidal anti-inflammatory drug (analgesic, anti-inflammatory, and antipyretic)

Used for: Treatment of moderately severe, acute pain, including post-operative pain and musculoskeletal strains or sprains.

How This Medication Works: Inhibits substances called prostaglandins that cause pain and inflammation.

Dosage Form and Strength:
- tablets (10 mg)
- injections (15 mg/mL, 30 mg/mL)

Storage:
- room temperature
- tightly closed
- protected from moisture and light

Administration:
- Usually taken 4 to 6 times daily.
- Do not lie down for at least 30 minutes after taking this medication.
- Take with food or milk if stomach upset occurs.
- Take with a full glass of water (6 to 8 ounces).

Precautions:
Do not use if:
- you are allergic to ibuprofen or any other nonsteroidal anti-inflammatory drug such as aspirin.

- medicine is beyond the expiration date or looks unusual in appearance.

Talk to your doctor if:

- you are taking aspirin; another nonsteroidal anti-inflammatory drug such as etodolac, indomethacin, or piroxicam; anticoagulants such as warfarin; steroids such as prednisone; lithium; diuretics such as furosemide and hydrochlorothiazide; methotrexate; beta blockers such as atenolol; or muscle relaxants.
- you have peptic ulcer disease, bleeding from your stomach or intestines, bleeding abnormalities, high blood pressure (hypertension), kidney disease, liver disease, heart disease, ulcerative colitis, asthma, nasal polyps, or a history of a stroke.
- you smoke tobacco or drink alcohol.

Side Effects:

Major:

- blood in stool or dark, tarry stool
- persistent or severe stomach or abdominal pain
- vomiting blood
- blood in urine or dark, smokey-colored urine
- difficulty urinating
- rash
- difficulty breathing
- swelling of the eyelids, throat, lips, or face
- vision or hearing changes
- unexplained sore throat or fever
- unusual bleeding or bruising
- irregular heartbeat

Minor:
- gas or heartburn
- diarrhea or constipation
- swelling of hands or feet
- dizziness or drowsiness
- headache

Time Required for Drug to Take Effect: Starts to relieve pain in 1 hour.

Symptoms of Overdose:
- stomach pain, nausea, or vomiting
- drowsiness or confusion
- headache
- loss of consciousness
- difficulty breathing
- heartburn

Special Notes:
- Alcohol may increase your risk of bleeding from the stomach or intestines while taking ketorolac.
- Tell the doctor or dentist you are taking ketorolac if you are going to have surgery or emergency treatment.
- Contact physician if pain or fever worsens.

labetalol

Brand Names:
Normodyne (Schering)
Trandate (Allen & Hansbury)

Generic Available: no

Type of Drug: antihypertensive (alpha- and beta-adrenergic blocking agent [alpha-, beta blocker])

Used for: Treatment of high blood pressure (hypertension)

How This Medication Works: Inhibits certain hormones that increase heart rate and blood pressure.

Dosage Form and Strength: tablets (100 mg, 200 mg, 300 mg)

Storage:
- room temperature
- protected from humidity

Administration:
- Usually taken once daily.
- Take labetalol at the same time every day.

Precautions:
Do not use if:
- you have ever had an allergic reaction to labetalol or another beta blocker such as atenolol or propranolol.

Talk to your doctor if:
- you are taking any other medications.

Side Effects:
Major:
- skin rash, itching
- sexual dysfunction
- difficulty breathing
- cold hands and feet
- confusion, hallucinations, nightmares

- palpitations or irregular heartbeat
- depression
- swelling of feet, ankles, or lower legs
- chest pressure or discomfort
- unusual bleeding or bruising
- dark urine
- yellow eyes or skin (jaundice)

Minor:
- tingling or numbness of the skin, especially the scalp
- low blood pressure (light-headedness, dizziness)
- drowsiness
- nervousness, anxiety, or trouble sleeping
- nausea, stomach upset, diarrhea, or constipation

Time Required for Drug to Take Effect: Starts
to work within 20 minutes to 2 hours, but it takes at least 2 to 4 weeks to see the maximal response.

Symptoms of Overdose:
- slow, fast, or irregular heartbeat
- fainting or severe dizziness
- difficulty breathing
- seizures or convulsions
- blue-tint to nail beds or palms

Special Notes:
- Do not discontinue without first talking with your doctor.
- Labetalol is not a cure, and you may have to take this medication for a long time.
- Changing positions slowly when sitting or standing up may help decrease dizziness caused by this medication.

- Older patients may also be more sensitive to cold temperatures while on this medication.
- Check with your physician or pharmacist before using any over-the-counter medications.
- Labetalol may slow the heart rate. Ask your doctor what your safe range is, but call your physician if your heart rate falls below 50 beats per minute.
- Be careful to avoid becoming dehydrated or over-heated. Avoid saunas and strenuous exercise in hot weather (especially during the hot summer months), and avoid alcoholic beverages. Drink plenty of fluids (at least 8 eight-ounce glasses daily) to prevent dehydration during exercise and hot weather.

leuprolide

Brand Names:
Lupron (TAP Pharmaceuticals)
Lupron Depot (TAP Pharmaceuticals)

Generic Available: no

Type of Drug: antineoplastic

Used for: Relief of symptoms of prostate cancer.

How This Medication Works: Decreases the levels of testosterone in the body.

Dosage Form and Strength: injection (5 mg/mL, 7.5 mg/mL)

Storage:
- room temperature
- protected from light

Administration:
- Usual doses are 1 mg daily by subcutaneous injection or 7.5 mg monthly by subcutaneous injection.
- Lupron Depot injections should be given by a doctor.

Precautions:
Do not use if:
- you have had an allergic reaction to leuprolide or gonadorelin.

Talk to your doctor if:
- you are taking any other medication.

Side Effects:
Major:
- chest pain or pressure
- leg pain or swelling
- shortness of breath

Minor:
- appetite decreased
- blurred vision
- bone pain
- breast swelling or tenderness
- constipation
- decrease in sexual desire or impotence
- dizziness
- swelling of the feet or lower legs
- headache

- hot flashes
- injection-site burning, itching, or redness
- nausea or vomiting
- numbness or tingling in the hands or feet

Time Required for Drug to Take Effect:
Becomes effective in 2 to 4 weeks.

Special Notes:
- Worsening of symptoms (bone pain, urination problems, weakness and tingling of the arms and legs) may occur in the first 1 to 2 weeks of therapy but should improve in 2 to 4 weeks.
- Do not discontinue without your doctor's consent.

levodopa and carbidopa combination
levodopa
carbidopa

Brand Names:
Levodopa/carbidopa combination:
Sinemet (DuPont)
Sinemet CR (DuPont)

Levodopa:
Dopar (Norwich Eaton)
Larodopa (Roche)
Carbidopa:
Lodosyn (Merck)

Generic Available: yes

Type of Drug: antiparkinsonian

Used for: Treatment of Parkinson disease, restless legs syndrome, and pain from shingles (herpes zoster infection).

How This Medication Works: Replaces the naturally occurring neurotransmitter dopamine, which is responsible for the coordination of movement.

Dosage Form and Strength:
Levodopa/carbidopa combination:
- tablets (10 mg/100 mg, 25 mg/100 mg, 25 mg/250 mg)
- controlled-release tablets (25 mg/100 mg, 50 mg/200 mg)

Levodopa:
- tablets (100 mg, 250 mg, 500 mg)
- capsules (250 mg, 500 mg)

Carbidopa:
- tablets (25 mg)

Storage:
- room temperature
- tightly closed

Administration:
Levodopa/carbidopa combination:
- Tablets initially taken 2 to 4 times daily depending on response, but may be increased to 8 or more tablets daily.
- Extended-release tablets initially taken 2 to 3 times daily depending on response, but may be increased to 8 tablets a day in divided doses.
- Extended-release tablets may be broken, but should not be crushed.

Levodopa:
- Dosing depends on individual patient.

Carbidopa:
- Dosing depends on individual patient, but total daily dose is usually not greater than 200 mg.

Precautions:

Do not use if:
- you have had an allergic response to levodopa, carbidopa, or tartrazine dye. (Certain tablets contain tartrazine. Check with your pharmacist.)
- you have melanoma (a type of skin cancer).

Talk to your doctor if:
- you have seizures, a history of peptic ulcers, heart disease, asthma, glaucoma, or mental disorders.
- you are taking metoclopramide, an antipsychotic (such as haloperidol or thioridazine), phenytoin, a monoamine oxidase (MAO) inhibitor (such as phenelzine or tranylcypromine, but not including selegiline), or vitamin B_6 (large doses).
- you drink alcohol on a regular or occasional basis.

Side Effects:

Major:
- palpitations
- fainting
- unusually high or low blood pressure
- chest pain
- urinary retention
- severe constipation with pain
- severe confusion
- severe or persistent nausea and vomiting

Minor:
- dizziness when sitting up or standing up
- decline in mood
- hallucinations
- abnormal movements (twisting or jerking spasms)
- stomach upset
- insomnia

Time Required for Drug to Take Effect: Starts
to work within days, but the maximum benefit may take
weeks.

Symptoms of Overdose:
- very high or very low blood pressure
- abnormal heart rhythm
- psychotic symptoms (hallucinations, delusions)
- severe constipation or abdominal pain
- unusual movements
- severe nausea or vomiting

Special Notes:
- Nausea or vomiting may occur when starting this
  medicine or when the dose is increased. Your
  doctor may recommend that you take the medicine with food or lower the dose until your body
  gets used to the medicine.
- Talk with your doctor before making changes in
  your regimen.
- Levodopa may cause a harmless darkening in the
  color of urine or sweat.
- Urine sugar tests may be altered by this medication.
- Response to levodopa may diminish over time,
  and doses may need to be increased.

- Patients sometimes develop abnormal body movements after taking this medication.
- Keep a record of the times when the medication is most effective and least effective. Good record keeping will help your doctor adjust your doses to get the maximum benefit for you.
- Keep a record of what you eat and your medication response. In some cases, certain types of food can interfere with medication absorption.

levothyroxine

Brand Names:
Levoxine (Daniels)　　　　Synthroid (Knoll)
Levothroid (Forest)

Generic Available: yes

Type of Drug: hormones (thyroid)

Used for: Treatment of low levels of thyroid hormone (hypothyroidism).

How This Medication Works: Increases low thyroid hormone levels to normal levels.

Dosage Form and Strength: tablets (12.5 µg, 25 µg, 50 µg, 75 µg, 100 µg, 112 µg, 125 µg, 150 µg, 175 µg, 200 µg, 300 µg)

Storage:
- room temperature
- tightly closed
- protected from light

Administration:
- Usual dosage is 75 to 100 µg once daily.
- The dosage will be adjusted monthly until the desired level of thyroid hormone is reached. (Doses usually start low and increase slowly to avoid side effects.)

Precautions:
Do not use if:
- you have had an allergic reaction to levothyroxine, thyroid hormone, thyroglobulin, liothyronine, or liotrix.
- you have hyperthyroidism.

Talk to your doctor if:
- you have heart disease (angina, chest pain, coronary artery disease, heart attack), diabetes, adrenocortical disease, pituitary disease, or malabsorption disease (celiac disease).
- you are taking any other medication, especially anticoagulants such as warfarin; diabetes medications such as insulin, glipizide, or tolbutamide; cholesterol medications such as lovastatin, cholestyramine, or niacin; digoxin; cough and cold medicines; seizure medications such as phenytoin, phenobarbital, or carbamazepine; cholestyramine; or colestipol.

Side Effects:
Major:
- hives or rash
- changes in appetite or weight loss
- chest pain
- diarrhea

- difficulty breathing
- fast or irregular heart beat
- hand tremor
- headache
- heat intolerance
- increased sweating
- irritability, nervousness, or insomnia
- leg cramps
- vomiting

Minor:
- clumsiness
- weakness
- increased sensitivity to cold
- constipation
- dry skin
- headache
- sleepiness or listlessness
- depression
- muscle aches
- weight gain

Time Required for Drug to Take Effect:
Usually takes 1 to 2 months to reach normal thyroid levels.

Symptoms of Overdose: Same as major side effects

Special Notes:
- Levothyroxine is not a cure and you may have to take this medication for a long time.
- Do not discontinue without first talking with your doctor.

lisinopril

Brand Names:
Prinivil (Stuart)
Zestril (Merck)

Generic Available: no

Type of Drug: antihypertensive (angiotensin-converting enzyme [ACE] inhibitor)

Used for: Treatment of high blood pressure (hypertension), congestive heart failure, and kidney disease caused by diabetes (diabetic nephropathy), and to preserve heart function after a heart attack.

How This Medication Works: Inhibits enzyme necessary for the formation of angiotensin, a substance that causes powerful constriction of blood vessels.

Dosage Form and Strength: tablets (2.5 mg, 5 mg, 10 mg, 20 mg, 40 mg)

Storage:
- room temperature
- tightly closed
- protected from humidity

Administration:
- Usually taken once daily.
- May be taken without regard to food.

Precautions:
Do not use if:
- you are allergic to lisinopril or other ACE inhibitors such as captopril or enalapril.

- you have liver disease (bilateral renal artery stenosis).

Talk to your doctor if:
- you are taking a diuretic (such as hydrochloroth-iazide or furosemide), a potassium supplement, indomethacin or any other nonsteroidal anti-inflammatory drug (such as aspirin, ibuprofen, naproxen, piroxicam, and ketoprofen), allop-urinol, digoxin, or lithium.

Side Effects:

Major:
- swelling of the mouth, lips, or tongue
- fainting
- generalized rash
- chest pain
- irregular heart beat

Minor:
- cough
- headache
- dizziness
- fatigue
- impotence
- decreased sexual desire

Time Required for Drug to Take Effect:

Usually starts to work after about 1 week of therapy, but sometimes several weeks of therapy are needed for it to reach its maximum effect.

Symptoms of Overdose:

- very low blood pressure
- profound muscle weakness
- nausea, vomiting, or diarrhea

Special Notes:
- Avoid salt substitutes containing potassium.
- You will need laboratory blood work while on lisinopril to monitor kidney function and electrolytes (sodium, potassium) in the blood.
- Avoid the use of aspirin or other nonsteroidal anti-inflammatory drugs such as ibuprofen and naproxen. Use acetaminophen for pain relief.
- Lisinopril may cause a dry cough. Talk to your doctor if it becomes particularly bothersome.

lithium

Brand Names:
Cibalith-S (Ciba-Geigy)   Lithonate (Reid-Rowell)
Eskalith (SK Beecham)   Lithotabs (Reid-Rowell)
Lithobid (Ciba-Geigy)   Lithane (Miles)

Generic Available: yes

Type of Drug: central nervous system drug

Used for: Treatment of manic depression (bipolar disorder).

How This Medication Works: Affects the transport of sodium and the activity of the neurotransmitters norepinephrine and serotonin.

Dosage Form and Strength:
- tablets (300 mg)
- extended-release tablets (300 mg, 450 mg)
- capsules (150 mg, 300 mg, 600 mg)
- oral syrup (approximately 300 mg/5 mL)

Storage:
- room temperature
- tightly closed

Administration:
- Swallow tablets, extended-release tablets, and capsules whole; do not crush or chew.
- Dilute oral syrup in juice.
- Take with meals or milk if stomach upset occurs.

Precautions:
Do not use if:
- you have had an allergic reaction to lithium.

Talk to your doctor if:
- you are taking any other medications, especially acetazolamide, carbamazepine, fluoxetine, haloperidol, loop diuretics (such as furosemide or bumetanide), methyldopa, nonsteroidal anti-inflammatory drugs (such as ibuprofen, etodolac or naproxen), theophylline, verapamil, or tricyclic antidepressants (such as amitriptyline or imipramine).
- you have kidney disease, seizures, diabetes, schizophrenia, or a history of leukemia.
- you experience diarrhea or fevers.

Side Effects:
Major:
- nausea
- vomiting
- diarrhea
- drowsiness
- muscle weakness
- severe trembling

Minor:
- increased frequency of urinaton
- nausea
- mild trembling of hands

Time Required for Drug to Take Effect: May require a week or longer before effects are evident.

Symptoms of Overdose:
- blurred vision
- clumsiness or confusion
- seizures
- dizziness
- severe trembling
- increase in amount of urine

Special Notes:
- This medication may cause drowsiness. Use caution when operating a motor vehicle or operating dangerous machinery.
- Drink at least eight 8-ounce glasses of fluids (water or juice) daily.

loratadine

Brand Name: Claritin (Schering)

Generic Available: no

Type of Drug: antihistamine

Used for: Treatment of allergies, hay fever, and hives.

How This Medication Works: Blocks histamine— a substance that causes sneezing, itching, and runny nose.

Dosage Form and Strength: tablets (10 mg)

Storage:
- room temperature
- protected from humidity

Administration:
- Take with full glass of water; drink plenty of fluids.
- Do not exceed the prescribed dose.
- Take with food or milk if stomach upset occurs.

Precautions:
Do not use if:
- you are allergic to loratadine or other antihistamines such as astemizole or diphenhydramine.
- you are taking erythromycin, ketoconazole, or itraconazole.
- you have severe liver disease.

Talk to your doctor if:
- you have asthma, difficulty breathing, liver disease, heart disease, high blood pressure, or an abnormal or irregular heartbeat.
- you are taking any medications, especially anti-infectives (such as ketoconazole, fluconazole, itraconazole, miconazole, metronidazole, or erythromycin), carbamazepine, and antidepressants.

Side Effects:
Major:
- skin rash, hives, or itching
- irregular heartbeat
- swelling of the mouth, lips, or face
- difficulty breathing
- yellowing of eyes or skin (jaundice)

Minor:
- hair loss
- cough
- menstrual disorders
- depression
- nightmares

Time Required for Drug to Take Effect: Starts
to work within 1 to 2 hours.

Symptoms of Overdose:
- irregular heartbeat
- seizures or convulsions
- drowsiness or dizziness
- dry mouth or throat
- trouble breathing
- trouble sleeping

Special Notes:
- Check with your physician and pharmacist before you use any over-the-counter medications.
- Tell the doctor you are taking loratadine before you have a skin test for allergies.
- Do not drink alcohol or take other medications that cause drowsiness or mental slowing.
- This medication may cause drowsiness. Do not operate a motor vehicle or other machinery while you are taking this medication.
- If you experience dryness of the mouth, try sugarless candy or gum, ice chips, or a saliva substitute.
- Tell the doctor or dentist you are taking this medication if you are going to have surgery or emergency treatment.

lorazepam

Brand Name: Ativan (Wyeth-Ayerst)

Generic Available: yes

Type of Drug: antianxiety

Used for: Treatment of anxiety.

How This Medication Works: Enhances the activity of the neurotransmitter gamma amino butyric acid to depress the central nervous system.

Dosage Form and Strength:
- tablets (0.5 mg, 1 mg, 2 mg)
- oral solution (2 mg/mL)

Storage:
- room temperature
- tightly closed
- protected from prolonged exposure to light

Administration:
- Usually taken 2 to 3 times daily.
- Take with food or milk if stomach upset occurs.

Precautions:
Do not use if:
- you have ever had an allergic reaction to lorazepam or other drugs in the benzodiazepine family such as diazepam or temazepam.

Talk to your doctor if:
- you are taking other medications that can depress the central nervous system such as alcohol, phenobarbital, or narcotics (such as codeine or meperidine).

- you have asthma, other lung problems, kidney disease, or liver disease.
- have been told that you snore.

Side Effects:

Major:
- confusion
- seizures
- hallucinations
- rash
- difficulty concentrating

Minor:
- unsteadiness or drowsiness
- slurred speech
- blurred vision

Time Required for Drug to Take Effect: Effects on anxiety may be seen within 2 hours.

Symptoms of Overdose:

- continuing confusion or slurred speech
- severe weakness or drowsiness
- shortness of breath
- seizures
- dry mouth
- increased heart rate
- tremors

Special Notes:

- Do not drink alcohol while taking this medication.
- Do not discontinue without your doctor's consent.
- If you notice dizziness, avoid activities requiring mental alertness, such as operating a motor vehicle or operating dangerous machinery.

losartan

Brand Name: Cozaar (Merck)

Generic Available: no

Type of Drug: antihypertensive (angiotensin II antagonist)

Used for: Treatment of high blood pressure (hypertension) and congestive heart failure.

How This Medication Works: Inhibits the formation of angiotensin, a substance that causes powerful constriction of blood vessels.

Dosage Form and Strength: tablets (25 mg, 50 mg)

Storage:
- room temperature
- tightly closed
- protected from humidity

Administration:
- Usually taken once or twice daily.
- May be taken without regard to food.

Precautions:
Do not use if:
- you are allergic to losartan.
- you have liver disease.

Talk to your doctor if:
- you are taking cimetidine, phenobarbital, or a diuretic such as hydrochlorothiazide.
- you have kidney disease.

Side Effects:

Major:
- unexplained or prolonged general tiredness
- swelling of the mouth, lips, or tongue

Minor:
- dizziness or blurred vision
- constipation
- dry mouth
- muscle pains and headache

Time Required for Drug to Take Effect:
Usually reaches its therapeutic effect in about 1 week.

Symptoms of Overdose
- very low blood pressure
- very rapid heart beat

Special Notes:
- Losartan is not a cure, and you may have to take this medication for a long time.

lovastatin

Brand Name: Mevacor (Merck)

Generic Available: no

Type of Drug: antihyperlipidemic

Used for: Treatment of high blood cholesterol levels and cardiovascular atherosclerosis.

How This Medication Works: Decreases the amount of cholesterol manufactured in the liver by inhibiting an enzyme.

Dosage Form and Strength: tablets (10 mg, 20 mg, 40 mg)

Storage:
- room temperature
- tightly closed
- protected from humidity

Administration:
- Usually administered once or twice daily.
- Take with meals. (If taking once daily, take with supper.)

Precautions:
Do not use if:
- you are allergic to lovastatin or similar drugs such as simvastatin, fluvastatin, or pravastatin.

Talk to your doctor if:
- you have liver disease.
- you are taking any other medication, especially cyclosporine, erythromycin, warfarin, niacin, or gemfibrozil.

Side Effects:
Major:
- unexplained muscle aches
- breathing difficulty
- swelling of the face, throat, lips, or tongue

Minor:
- insomnia
- abdominal pain, cramps, or diarrhea
- headache
- dizziness
- taste disturbance

Time Required for Drug to Take Effect: Starts lowering blood cholesterol levels in 1 to 2 weeks, but it may take 4 to 6 weeks to reach maximum effectiveness.

Symptoms of Overdose: no specific symptoms

Special Notes:
- After beginning lovastatin therapy, your doctor will recheck your cholesterol levels in 1 to 3 months.
- Use a sunblock with at least SPF 15 when outside because lovastatin may increase your sensitivity to the sun.
- Do not drink alcohol while taking this medication.
- Reduce your dietary cholesterol.
- Lovastatin is not a cure and must be taken on a long-term basis to have an effect.
- Your doctor will monitor your liver function with laboratory blood work while you are on this medicine.

meclizine

Brand Names:

Antivert (Roerig)

Antrizine (Major)

Ru-Vert-M (Reid-Rowell)

Bonine (Leeming)

Dizmiss (JMI Canton)

Meni-D (Seatrace)

Generic Available: yes

Type of Drug: antiemetic/antivertigo

Used for: Treatment of motion sickness and vertigo associated with inner-ear problems.

How This Medication Works: Decreases the sensitivity of the inner ear to motion and sensitivity of the vomit center to messages arriving from the inner ear.

Dosage Forms and Strength:
- tablets (12.5 mg, 25 mg, 50 mg)
- chewable tablets (25 mg)
- capsules (25 mg)

Storage:
- room temperature
- tightly closed

Administration:
- For motion sickness, take 1 tablet 1 hour before leaving on trip and once daily during travel.
- For dizziness, take 1 tablet 2 to 3 times daily.

Precautions:
Do not use if:
- you have ever had an allergic reaction to meclizine.
- you have glaucoma, colitis, severe constipation, prostate problems, or myasthenia gravis.

Talk to your doctor if:
- you are taking medicines for irregular heartbeat, Parkinson disease, upset stomach or cramping, hiatal hernia, allergies, anxiety, depression, sleep problems, hallucinations, or other mental conditions.
- you have severe dry mouth, constipation, urinary retention, or breathing problems.
- you are taking metoclopramide, antipsychotics (such as chlorpromazine or haloperidol), tricyclic

antidepressants (such as amitriptyline, imipramine, or nortriptyline), muscle relaxants, or prescription pain medicines.

Side Effects:

Major:
- eye pain
- dilated pupils
- severe constipation
- difficult or painful urination
- seizures
- severe agitation or confusion
- hot, dry, flushed skin
- fever

Minor:
- dizziness, drowsiness, or sedation
- dry mouth
- blurred vision
- mild constipation

Time Required for Drug to Take Effect: Starts to work in 30 to 60 minutes.

Symptoms of Overdose:
- eye pain
- dilated pupils
- severe constipation
- inability to urinate
- seizures
- severe confusion, agitation, or psychosis
- hyperactivity, combativeness
- hot, dry flushed skin, fever
- severe muscle weakness or cramping
- coma, stupor

Special Notes:
- In general, older adults are more sensitive to the side effects of this medicine; ask your doctor or pharmacist to recommend the lowest dose that will be effective.
- Do not drink alcohol while taking this medication.
- Avoid staying out in hot weather for long periods.

medroxyprogesterone

Brand Names:
Amen (Carnrick)　　　　Curretab (Solvay)
Cycrin (ESI Pharma)　　Provera (Upjohn)

Generic Available: yes

Type of Drug: hormone

Used for: Prevention of endometrial changes from estrogen replacement therapy, hormone imbalances, and endometriosis.

How This Medication Works: Prevents overgrowth of the endometrium caused by estrogen replacement therapy. Normalizes hormone levels in other conditions.

Dosage Form and Strength: tablets (2.5 mg, 5 mg, 10 mg)

Storage:
- room temperature
- tightly closed
- protected from light

Administration:
- When used with estrogen, the usual dose is 2.5 mg daily or 5 mg on days 15 through 28 in every 28-day cycle.

Precautions:
Do not use if:
- you have had an allergic reaction to medroxy-progesterone, hydroxyprogesterone, megestrol, norethindrone, norgestrel, or progesterone.
- you have breast cancer, liver disease, or abnormal vaginal bleeding.

Talk to your doctor if:
- you have blood clots (thrombophlebitis).
- you are taking any other medication, especially bromocriptine.

Side Effects:
Major:
- breast tenderness or chest pain
- depression
- fainting or sudden, severe headache
- hair loss
- leg pain or swelling
- menstrual bleeding changes
- rash
- slurred speech
- rapid weight gain
- yellowing of the eyes or skin (jaundice)

Minor:
- acne
- dizziness or headache
- gum changes (tenderness, swelling, or pain)

- hair growth
- nausea and vomiting
- sun sensitivity

Time Required for Drug to Take Effect: Varies depending on condition being treated.

Symptoms of Overdose: none known

Special Notes:
- Regular brushing and flossing is necessary to help prevent gum side effects.
- Use a sunblock with at least SPF 15 when outside because medroxyprogesterone may increase your sensitivity to the sun.
- PremPro and PremPhase are combinations of estrogen and medroxyprogesterone; see profile on estrogen for more information.

meperidine

Brand Name: Demerol (Winthrop)

Generic Available: yes

Type of Drug: analgesic

Used for: Relief of moderate to severe pain.

How This Medication Works: Decreases the central nervous system's recognition of pain impulses.

Dosage Form and Strength:
- tablets (50 mg, 100 mg)
- syrup (50 mg/5 mL)

Storage:
- room temperature
- protected from humidity

Administration:
- Do not exceed the maximum number of doses per day. Never take more tablets per dose than your doctor has prescribed.
- Take with food or milk if stomach upset occurs.
- Take each dose of the syrup in at least a half glass of water.

Precautions:
Do not use if:
- you are allergic to meperidine or related drugs such as fentanyl, loperamide, or diphenoxylate.
- you are taking a monoamine oxidase (MAO) inhibitor such as phenelzine or tranylcypromine or have taken one within 14 days.

Talk to your doctor if:
- you have substance abuse problems or alcoholism; brain disease or head injury; colitis; seizures; emotional problems or mental illness; emphysema, asthma, or other lung diseases; kidney, liver, or thyroid disease; prostate problems or problems with urination; or gallbladder disease or gallstones.
- you are taking any other medications, especially phenytoin, naltrexone, and medications that can cause drowsiness, such as antihistamines, barbiturates (phenobarbital), benzodiazepines (diazepam, alprazolam, lorazepam), muscle relaxants, or antidepressants.

Side Effects:

Major:
- skin rash or hives
- fainting
- severe confusion or hallucinations
- painful or difficult urination
- frequent urge to urinate
- fast, slow, or pounding heart beat
- seizures, tremors, or uncontrolled movements
- irregular or difficult breathing
- depression

Minor:
- constipation
- drowsiness
- dry mouth
- general feeling of discomfort or illness
- loss of appetite
- nervousness, restlessness, or insomnia

Time Required for Drug to Take Effect: Starts to work within 10 to 15 minutes and continues to relieve pain for 2 to 4 hours.

Symptoms of Overdose:
- cold, clammy skin
- seizures
- diarrhea
- stomach cramps or pain
- severe dizziness, drowsiness, or confusion
- continued nausea or vomiting
- severe nervousness or restlessness
- difficulty breathing
- slowed heartbeat

Special Notes:

- This medication may make you drowsy and dizzy. Do not operate a motor vehicle or other machinery while you are taking this medication.
- Meperidine may cause constipation. This side effect may be diminished by drinking 6 to 8 full glasses of water each day. Increase fresh fruit in your diet. If using this medication for chronic pain, ask your doctor about adding a stool softener–laxative combination.
- Check with your physician or pharmacist before using any over-the-counter medications.
- When meperidine is used over a long period of time, your body may become tolerant and require larger doses. If your pain is no longer relieved by the current dose, talk to your doctor or pharmacist.
- Do not stop taking this medication abruptly.
- Nausea and vomiting may occur after the first few doses; this effect will diminish with time.
- Do not drink alcohol while taking this medication.
- If you experience dry mouth, try sugarless candy or gum, ice chips, or a saliva substitute.
- Use this medication as prescribed; do not exceed the dose or frequency prescribed by your doctor.

metaproterenol

Brand Names:

Alupent (Boehringer-Ingelheim)
Metaprel (Sandoz)

Generic Available: yes

Type of Drug: bronchodilator

Used for: Treatment of asthma.

How This Medication Works: Causes the passageways in the lungs to dilate.

Dosage Form and Strength:
- tablets (10 mg, 20 mg)
- syrup (10 mg/5 mL)
- inhaler (0.65 mg/inhalation)

Storage:
- room temperature
- protected from humidity

Administration:
- Have your doctor or pharmacist demonstrate the proper procedure for using your inhaler, and make sure they have you practice your technique in front of them.
- Allow at least 2 minutes between inhalations (puffs).
- If you have more than one inhaler, it is important to administer your inhalers in the correct order. If you are using metaproterenol and another inhaler, such as ipratropium or beclomethasone, use the metaproterenol first. Wait at least 5 minutes before inhaling the second medication.

Precautions:
Do not use if:
- you have had an allergic reaction to metaproterenol, albuterol, epinephrine, salmeterol, or terbutaline.

Talk to your doctor if:
- you have diabetes, heart disease, high blood pressure (hypertension), problems with circulation or blood vessels, seizures, convulsions, or thyroid disease.
- you are taking any other medications, especially medications for heart disease, high blood pressure (hypertension), migraine headaches, or depression.

Side Effects:
Major:
- skin rash, itching, or hives
- wheezing or difficulty breathing
- bluish coloring of your skin
- swelling of face, lips, or eyelids
- fainting or dizziness
- chest discomfort or pressure
- irregular heartbeat
- numbness or tingling in hands or feet
- hallucinations

Minor:
- nervousness, tremor, or trembling
- coughing
- dryness or irritation of mouth or throat
- unpleasant taste
- flushing or redness of the face
- headache
- increased sweating
- muscle cramps or twitching
- nausea or vomiting
- trouble sleeping
- drowsiness

Time Required for Drug to Take Effect:

Inhaled medications start to work within 60 seconds; tablets take about 15 minutes.

Symptoms of Overdose:

- chest discomfort or pressure
- chills, fever, seizures, or convulsions
- irregular heartbeat
- severe nausea or vomiting
- severe trouble breathing
- severe tremor or trembling
- blurred vision
- unusual paleness and coldness of skin

Special Notes:

- Sometimes a spacer device is used with your inhaler. A spacer device helps the medication get to the lungs instead of the mouth or throat.
- Check with your physician and pharmacist before using any other medication.
- Save the applicator from your inhaler. There may be refills that fit into your applicator.
- Keep track of how many inhalations are left and get your medication refilled about 1 week before you expect to run out.

metformin

Brand Name: Glucophage (Bristol-Myers-Squibb)

Generic Available: no

Type of Drug: hormone (antidiabetic)

Used for: Lowering glucose levels in type II (non–insulin-dependent or adult-onset) diabetes.

How This Medication Works: The exact mechanism is unknown, but it appears that metformin increases the sensitivity of cells to insulin.

Dosage Form and Strength: tablets (500 mg, 850 mg)

Storage:
- room temperature
- tightly closed
- protected from humidity

Administration:
- Usually taken 2 or 3 times daily.
- May be taken without regard to meals.
- Take with food if stomach upset occurs.
- Individual dosage will vary, depending on glycemic control and response to the medication. (Total daily dose should not exceed 2,550 mg.)

Precautions:
Do not use if:
- you are allergic to metformin.
- medicine is beyond the expiration date.
- you are taking tetracycline.

Talk to your doctor if:
- you have kidney disease, respiratory disease, heart disease, or pancreatitis.
- you have ever had liver disease or diabetic ketoacidosis.
- you have been told you have type I (insulin-dependent or juvenile-onset) diabetes.

- you consume more than 2 alcoholic drinks on a daily basis.
- you are taking cimetidine, ranitidine, trimethoprim, nifedipine, furosemide, or procainamide.

Side Effects:

Major:
- hypoglycemia (sweating, shaking, headache, irritability, blurred vision, seizures, and coma)
- persistent diarrhea, vomiting, or stomach upset
- malaise, increasing sleepiness
- unexplained muscle aches or cramps
- painful, swollen tongue

Minor:
- nausea or vomiting
- diarrhea
- loss of appetite
- bloatedness

Time Required for Drug to Take Effect:

Begins to work in about 3 hours and reaches its maximum effectiveness in 1 or 2 days.

Symptoms of Overdose:

- profound hypoglycemia
- seizures
- coma

Special Notes:

- Do not drink alcohol while taking this medication.
- Do not discontinue without first talking with your doctor.
- Talk to your doctor or diabetes educator about how to handle sick days.

- When you begin metformin therapy, check your blood glucose level frequently, right before meals or 2 hours after you have eaten.
- Metformin can be used alone or in combination with an oral antidiabetic agent in the sulfonylurea class such as glyburide or glipizide.
- Side effects should disappear with continued use.
- Metformin can cause a vitamin B_{12} deficiency and a rare but very serious side effect called lactic acidosis. For these reasons, your doctor will take blood tests to monitor your blood count and kidney function.
- The use of metformin to reduce insulin requirements in type I (insulin-dependent or juvenile-onset) diabetes is controversial and is considered investigational at this time.
- Tell the doctor or dentist you are taking metformin if you are going to have surgery or emergency treatment.

methotrexate

Brand Name: Rheumatrex (Lederle)

Generic Available: yes

Type of Drug: antirheumatic

Used for: Treatment of rheumatoid arthritis.

How This Medication Works: Blocks the production of white blood cells which are, in part, responsible for inflammation.

Dosage Form and Strength: tablets (2.5 mg)
Storage:
- room temperature
- tightly closed

Administration:
- Usually taken either as a single dose (3 tablets) once a week or 1 or 2 tablets every 12 hours for 2 or 3 doses each week.

Precautions:
Do not use if:
- you have ever had an allergic reaction to methotrexate.

Talk to your doctor if:
- you have liver problems, kidney problems, an infection, or anemia.
- you have ever had an ulcer, bowel disease, cancer, or problems that affect your immune system.
- you have taken cancer medication.
- you are taking pain relievers, blood thinners, folic acid, or probenecid.

Side Effects:
Major:
- severe stomach pain or diarrhea
- bleeding
- infection
- dry cough or breathing problems
- rash
- back pain
- problems with urination
- seizures

- change in vision
- mouth sores or ulcers

Minor:
- dizziness or drowsiness
- headache
- hair loss

Time Required for Drug to Take Effect:
Becomes effective in 1 to 2 months.

Symptoms of Overdose:
- severe stomach pain, vomiting, or diarrhea
- bleeding or easy bruising
- seizures
- unusual drowsiness or weakness

Special Notes:
- If you are planning to get a vaccination, inform the doctor that you are taking this medicine.
- You will be required to have blood tests and possibly other tests while taking this medicine.

methyldopa

Brand Name: Aldomet (Merck)

Generic Available: yes

Type of Drug: antihypertensive

Used for: Treatment of high blood pressure (hypertension).

How This Medication Works: Acts on the central nervous system to dilate blood vessels.

Dosage Form and Strength:
- tablets (125 mg, 250 mg, 500 mg)
- liquid/oral suspension (250 mg/5 mL)

Storage:
- room temperature
- tightly closed
- protected from humidity

Administration:
- Usually taken 3 times daily.
- May be taken without regard to food.
- For liquid, shake bottle well before pouring.

Precautions:
Do not use if:
- you are allergic to methyldopa.
- you have liver disease.

Talk to your doctor if:
- you have kidney disease.
- you are taking haloperidol, levodopa, lithium, propranolol, or tolbutamide.
- you are allergic to sulfites.

Side Effects:
Major:
- yellow pigment in skin (jaundice)
- chest pain
- unexplained prolonged general tiredness

Minor:
- sedation
- impotence
- urine discoloration
- nausea and vomiting

- headache
- weight gain
- dry mouth

Time Required for Drug to Take Effect: Has
its full effect in about 2 days.

Symptoms of Overdose
- sedation or coma
- weakness
- slow heart beat (less than 50 beats per minute)

Special Notes:
- Tell your doctor that you are taking methyldopa before having any blood or urine tests done.
- Do not discontinue without your doctor's consent.
- Your doctor will monitor your liver function and blood cell count while you are on methyldopa.
- If you experience dryness of the mouth, try sugarless candy or gum, ice chips, or a saliva substitute.
- Tell the doctor or dentist you are taking this medication before any treatment.
- Methyldopa is not a cure, and you may have to take this medication for a long time.

methylphenidate

Brand Names:
Ritalin (Ciba-Geigy)
Ritalin-SR (Ciba-Geigy)

Generic Available: yes

Type of Drug: stimulant

Used for: Treatment of attention-deficit hyperactivity disorder and narcolepsy.

How This Medication Works: Stimulates the central nervous system to decrease sensation of tiredness.

Dosage Form and Strength:
- tablets (5 mg, 10 mg, 20 mg)
- extended-release tablets (20 mg)

Storage:
- room temperature
- tightly closed

Administration:
- Tablets usually taken 2 to 3 times daily (1 to 3 times daily for extended-release tablets).
- Swallow extended-release tablets whole.
- Take with food.

Precautions:
Do not use if:
- you are allergic to methylphenidate.

Talk to your doctor if:
- you are taking any other medications, especially guanethidine and monamine oxidase (MAO) inhibitors such as phenelzine or tranylcypromine.
- you have seizures, high blood pressure (hypertension), glaucoma, severe anxiety, or depression.

Side Effects:
Major:
- increased heart rate
- mood changes
- weight loss

Minor:
- decreased appetite
- difficulty sleeping
- headache
- nausea and vomiting
- drowsiness

Time Required for Drug to Take Effect: Effects seen within a few hours.

Symptoms of Overdose:
- confusion
- seizures or tremors
- dry mouth
- increased heart rate
- vomiting

Special Notes:
- Do not discontinue without first talking with your doctor.
- If you have difficulty sleeping, take last dose of day before 6 P.M.

methylprednisolone

Brand Name: Medrol (Upjohn)

Generic Available: yes

Type of Drug: hormone (adrenal cortical steroid)

Used for: Treatment of rheumatoid arthritis, lung diseases, lupus, ulcerative colitis, eye disorders, skin problems, poison ivy, and some cancers.

How This Medication Works: Methylpredniso-lone is a cortisonelike substance produced in the body. In most conditions, its mechanism is unknown, but often the benefits are from decreasing inflammation.

Dosage Form and Strength: tablets (2 mg, 4 mg, 8 mg, 16 mg, 32 mg)

Storage:
- room temperature
- tightly closed
- protected from light

Administration:
- The dosage of methylprednisolone varies from person to person, depending on disease treated.
- If you are taking methylprednisolone once daily, take it before 9:00 A.M.
- Take with food or milk if stomach upset occurs.
- If you miss a dose and you are taking it more than once daily, take the dose as soon as you remember it; if you do not remember until the next dose, double the dose and return to your regular schedule. If you are taking the dose once daily, take the dose as soon as you remember it unless it is the next day; if it is the next day, take your regular dose and return to your regular schedule; do not double the dose. If you miss a dose taking it every other day, take the dose as soon as you remember it that day; if it is the day after the dose was to be taken, take it and start over on the every-other-day schedule, skipping the next day and taking it the following day. If you miss more than one dose, call your doctor.

Precautions:

Do not use if:

- you have had an allergic reaction to methylpredisolone, dexamethasone, predaisolone, prednisolone, prednisone, cortisone, hydrocortisone, triamclolone, or any other steroids

Talk to your doctor if:

- you have bone disease, diabetes, emotional problems, glaucoma, fungal infections, heart disease, high blood pressure (hypertension), high cholesterol, kidney disease, liver disease, myasthenia gravis, stomach problems (ulcers or gastritis), thyroid disease, tuberculosis, or ulcerative colitis.
- you are taking any other medication, especially aspirin or nonsteroidal anti-inflammatory drugs (ibuprofen, indomethacin), anticoagulants (warfarin), cholestyramine, colestipol, diabetes medications (insulin, glipizide, tolbutamide), diuretics (hydrochlorothiazide, furosemide), seizure medications (phenobarbital, phenytoin), or tuberculosis medications (isoniazid, rifampin).

Side Effects:

Major:

- acne or other skin problems
- back or rib pain
- unusual bleeding or bruising
- bloody or black, tarry stools
- eye pain or blurred vision
- fever and headaches
- slow wound healing
- mood changes
- muscle weakness or wasting

- rapid weight gain (3 to 5 pounds in a week)
- seizures
- shortness of breath
- sore throat
- stomach pain or enlargement
- increased thirst and urination

Minor:
- dizziness
- increased appetite
- indigestion
- increased sweating or blushing
- restlessness and sleep disorders

Time Required for Drug to Take Effect: Varies depending on the condition treated.

Symptoms of Overdose:
- agitation
- mania or psychotic behavior

Special Notes:
- Methylprednisolone can cause low potassium levels. Orange juice and bananas can replace some potassium. Talk to your doctor before making diet changes.
- If you take methylprednisolone longer than 1 week, the dosage may need adjustments during stressful times. Tell your doctor if you have an infection or injury or if you have to have surgery.
- If you take methylprednisolone for long periods, it may cause glaucoma, cataracts, high blood sugar, and diabetes.
- While taking methylprednisolone, you should not receive live vaccinations or immunizations.

metoclopramide

Brand Names:
Maxolon (SK Beecham)
Reglan (Robins)

Generic Available: yes

Type of Drug: antiemetic/antivertigo

Used for: Treatment of nausea and vomiting (especially with cancer chemotherapy), stomach problems in diabetes, and heartburn (gastroesophageal reflux disease [GERD]).

How This Medication Works: Increases the movement (muscle contractions) inside the stomach and intestines and inhibits the nausea center in the brain.

Dosage Form and Strength:
- tablets (5 mg, 10 mg)
- syrup (5 mg/5 mL)

Storage:
- room temperature
- protected from humidity

Administration:
- Take 30 minutes before meals and at bedtime.

Precautions:
Do not use if:
- you are allergic to metoclopramide.

Talk to your doctor if:
- you have bleeding from stomach or intestines, disorders of stomach or intestines, Parkinson

disease, epilepsy or seizures, kidney disease, or liver disease.
- you are taking any other medications, especially medications that may make you drowsy such as antihistamines, cold medications, sedatives, tranquilizers, sleeping medications, pain relievers, seizure medications, and muscle relaxants.

Side Effects:

Major:
- skin rash, hives, or itching
- shuffling walk
- trembling of hands
- chills, fever, or sore throat
- difficulty speaking or swallowing
- masklike face
- stiffness

Minor:
- drowsiness
- restlessness and irritabiliy
- breast tenderness or swelling
- constipation or diarrhea
- depression
- headache
- nausea
- trouble sleeping
- unusual dryness of the mouth

Time Required for Drug to Take Effect: Starts to work within 30 to 60 minutes.

Symptoms of Overdose:
- confusion
- drowsiness

Special Notes:
- Check with your physician or pharmacist before using any over-the-counter medications.
- This medication may cause drowsiness. Use caution when operating a motor vehicle or operating dangerous machinery.
- Do not drink alcohol while taking this medication.
- Metoclopramide may worsen the symptoms of Parkinson disease.
- If you experience dryness of the mouth, try sugarless candy or gum, ice chips, or a saliva substitute.

metolazone

Brand Names:
Zaroxolyn (Fisons)
Mykrox (Fisons)

Generic Available: no

Type of Drug: diuretic

Used for: Treatment of fluid retention (edema) and high blood pressure (hypertension), prevention of calcium kidney stones, and enhancement of other diuretics' effectiveness.

How This Medication Works: Increases the amount of sodium and chloride excretion in the kidney, resulting in loss of water through urine.

Dosage Form and Strength: tablets (0.5 mg, 2.5 mg, 5 mg, 10 mg)

Storage:
- room temperature
- tightly closed
- protected from humidity

Administration:
- Usually taken once daily, in the morning.
- If also taking furosemide or bumetanide, take metolazone 30 minutes before you take furosemide or bumetanide.
- Take with food or milk if stomach upset occurs.

Precautions:
Do not use if:
- you are allergic to metolazone or other thiazide diuretics such as hydrochlorothiazide or chlorthalidone.
- you are allergic to other sulfa drugs such as oral diabetes medication (such as tolazamide, glipizide, or glyburide), acetazolamide, loop diuretics (such as furosemide or bumetanide), or sulfa antibacterial medication (sulfamethoxazole or sulfasalazine).

Talk to your doctor if:
- you have liver disease, kidney disease, or gout.
- you are taking allopurinol, warfarin, calcium supplements, digoxin, lithium, loop diuretics (such as furosemide, bumetanide, or torsemide), methyldopa, oral diabetes medication (such as tolazamide, glipizide, or glyburide), insulin, vitamin D, cholestyramine, or nonsteroidal anti-inflammatory drugs (such as ibuprofen, sulindac, indomethacin, or diclofenac).

Side Effects:
Major:
- seizures
- chest pain
- prolonged vomiting or diarrhea
- unexplained muscle pain, weakness, or cramps

Minor:
- headache
- dry mouth
- dizziness or drowsiness

Time Required for Drug to Take Effect:
Begins to exert its diuretic effect within 1 hour.

Symptoms of Overdose
- dizziness, drowsiness, lethargy, fainting, or coma
- confusion
- muscular weakness
- nausea and vomiting

Special Notes:
- Your doctor will monitor therapy with regular blood tests.
- Take with orange juice or a banana to help replace lost potassium.
- Unless otherwise instructed by your doctor, it is important to drink 6 to 8 eight-ounce glasses of water daily to avoid dehydration.
- Use a sunblock with at least SPF 15 when outside because metolazone may increase your sensitivity to the sun.
- If you experience dryness of the mouth, try sugarless candy or gum, ice chips or a saliva substitute.

- Weigh yourself daily. If you gain or lose more than 1 pound per day, call your doctor.
- Changing positions slowly when sitting and/or standing up may help decrease dizziness caused by this medication.
- If you have diabetes, you may need to check your blood glucose more frequently.
- You will need to have blood tests done periodically during therapy.

metoprolol

Brand Names:
Lopressor (Ciba-Geigy)
Toprol XL (Astra)

Generic Available: no

Type of Drug: antihypertensive (beta-adrenergic blocking agent [beta blocker])

Used for: Relief of angina (chest pressure or discomfort) and treatment of high blood pressure (hypertension) and heart attacks.

How This Medication Works: Inhibits certain hormones that increase heart rate and blood pressure.

Dosage Form and Strength: tablets (50 mg, 100 mg, 200 mg)

Storage:
- room temperature
- protected from humidity

Administration:
- For high blood pressure (hypertension) and angina, usually taken once daily.
- Take at the same time every day.
- Administration in cases of heart attack limited to hospital use.

Precautions:
Do not use if:
- you have ever had an allergic reaction to metoprolol or another beta blocker such as atenolol or propranolol.

Talk to your doctor if:
- you are taking any other medication, especially medication for diabetes, asthma, high blood pressure (hypertension), heart disease, or depression.
- you have asthma, hay fever, allergies, hives, eczema, breathing problems (such as emphysema or chronic bronchitis), slow heart rate, heart disease, problems with circulation or your blood vessels, diabetes or problems with your blood sugar, kidney disease, liver disease, thyroid disease, or a history of depression.

Side Effects:
Major:
- skin rash, itching
- sexual dysfunction
- difficulty breathing
- cold hands and feet
- confusion, hallucinations, nightmares
- palpitations or irregular heart beat
- depression

- swelling of feet, ankles, or lower legs
- chest pressure or discomfort
- unusual bleeding or bruising

Minor:
- nervousness, anxiety, and trouble sleeping
- light-headedness, dizziness, and drowsiness
- nausea, stomach upset, diarrhea, or constipation

Time Required for Drug to Take Effect: Starts
to work within 1.5 to 4 hours, but it takes at least 2 to 4 weeks to see the maximal response.

Symptoms of Overdose:
- slow, fast, or irregular heart beat
- fainting or severe dizziness
- difficulty breathing
- seizures or convulsions
- blue tint to nail beds or palms

Special Notes:
- Do not stop taking metoprolol without first consulting with your doctor.
- Metoprolol is not a cure and you may have to take this medication for a long time.
- Check with your physician or pharmacist before using any over-the-counter medications.
- Older patients may be more sensitive to cold temperatures while taking metoprolol.
- If you notice dizziness, avoid activities requiring mental alertness, such as operating a motor vehicle or operating dangerous machinery.
- Changing positions slowly when sitting and/or standing up may help decrease dizziness caused by this medication.

- Metoprolol is used to prevent angina, and sublingual tablets (those placed under the tongue) may be required to treat an acute attack of angina.
- Metoprolol may slow the heart rate. Ask your doctor what your safe range is, but call your physician if your heart rate falls below 50 beats per minute.
- Be careful to avoid becoming dehydrated or overheated. Avoid saunas, strenuous exercise in hot weather, especially during the hot summer months, and avoid alcoholic beverages. Drink plenty of fluids to prevent dehydration during exercise and hot weather.

metronidazole

Brand Names:
Flagyl (Searle)
Protostat (Ortho)

Generic Available: yes

Type of Drug: anti-infective

Used for: Treatment of infections of the blood, skin, vagina, bone, and respiratory tract caused by susceptible bacteria or protozoa, and treatment of Crohn disease.

How This Medication Works: Appears to enter invading organisms and stop DNA synthesis.

Dosage Form and Strength: tablets (250 mg, 500 mg)

Storage:
- room temperature
- tightly closed
- protected from humidity

Administration:
- Usually taken 3 to 4 times daily.
- Take at even intervals.
- Take with food to avoid stomach upset.
- Take until completely gone, even if symptoms have improved.

Precautions:
Do not use if:
- you are allergic to metronidazole.
- medicine is beyond the expiration date.

Talk to your doctor if:
- you have ever had liver disease.
- you are taking phenobarbital, warfarin, disulfiram, phenytoin, or lithium.

Side Effects:
Major:
- numbness or tingling (pins and needles) of the hands or feet
- seizures
- rash

Minor:
- metallic taste
- darkening of the urine (deep red-brown in color)
- dizziness
- stomach upset
- headache

Time Required for Drug to Take Effect:
Begins to kill infecting organisms within hours after first dose. However, you must continue to take the drug for the full course of treatment, even if symptoms disappear.

Symptoms of Overdose:
- nausea and vomiting
- staggering
- seizures

Special Notes:
- Do not drink alcohol while taking this medication.
- Take until completely gone, even if symptoms have improved.
- Do not use for infections other than the one for which it was prescribed.

misoprostol

Brand Name: Cytotec (Searle)

Generic Available: no

Type of Drug: gastrointestinal (prostaglandin)

Used for: Prevention of ulcers induced by non-steroidal anti-inflammatory drugs.

How This Medication Works: Replaces prosta-glandins lost because of nonsteroidal anti-inflammatory drug therapy.

Dosage Form and Strength: tablets (100 µg, 200 µg)

Storage:
- room temperature
- protected from humidity

Administration:
- Take after food if stomach upset occurs.

Precautions:
Do not use if:
- you are allergic to misoprostol.

Talk to your doctor if:
- you have epilepsy, seizures, or blood vessel disease.
- you are taking any other medications.

Side Effects:
Major:
- vaginal bleeding

Minor:
- abdominal cramping, diarrhea, or constipation
- headache
- nausea or vomiting

Time Required for Drug to Take Effect: Starts to work within 15 to 30 minutes. However, for preventive effect, it must already be ingested when you take the nonsteroidal anti-inflammatory drugs.

Symptoms of Overdose:
- sedation
- tremor, convulsions, or seizures
- difficulty breathing
- light-headedness
- irregular heartbeat
- abdominal pain

Special Notes:
- Check with your physician or pharmacist before using any over-the-counter medications.
- Side effects should disappear with continued use.
- Avoid magnesium-containing antacids.

morphine

Brand Names:
MS Contin (Purdue-
  Frederick)
MSIR (Purdue-Frederick)
Oramorph SR (Roxane)

RMS (Upsher-Smith)
Roxanol (Roxane)
Roxanol SR (Roxane)

Generic Available:
- tablets, soluble tablets, capsules, liquid, rectal suppositories: yes
- sustained-release tablets: no

Type of Drug: analgesic

Used for: Relief of moderate to severe pain and shortness of breath due to heart or lung disease.

How This Medication Works: Acts in the central nervous system to decrease the recognition of pain impulses.

Dosage Form and Strength:
- tablets (15 mg, 30 mg)
- soluble tablets (10 mg, 15 mg, 30 mg)
- sustained-release tablets (15 mg, 30 mg, 60 mg, 100 mg)
- capsules (15 mg, 30 mg)

- liquid (10 mg/5 mL, 20 mg/5 mL, 20 mg/mL, 100 mg/5 mL)
- rectal suppositories (5 mg, 10 mg, 20 mg, 30 mg)

Storage:
- room temperature
- protected from humidity

Administration:
- Tablets, capsules, solution, and suppositories are usually taken every 4 hours.
- Sustained-release tablets are usually taken every 12 hours.
- Dosage is individualized for each patient, depending on the pain and previous exposure to morphine.
- Never take more tablets per dose or more doses per day than your doctor has prescribed.
- Take with milk or food if stomach upset occurs.
- Do not crush or chew sustained-release tablet.

Precautions:
Do not use if:
- you are allergic to morphine or other narcotics such as hydrocodone, codeine, hydromorphone, or oxycodone.

Talk to your doctor if:
- you have alcoholism or other substance abuse problems; brain disease or head injury; colitis; seizures; emotional problems or mental illness; emphysema, asthma, or other lung diseases; kidney, liver, or thyroid disease; prostate problems or problems with urination; or gallbladder disease or gallstones.

- you are taking naltrexone, zidovudine, or any other medications, especially those that can cause drowsiness such as antihistamines, barbiturates (such as phenobarbital), benzodiazepines (diazepam, alprazolam, lorazepam), muscle relaxants, or antidepressants.

Side Effects:
Major:
- skin rash or hives
- severe confusion or hallucinations
- fainting
- irregular difficult breathing
- painful or difficult urination
- frequent urge to urinate
- fast, slow, or pounding heart beat
- depression
- trembling or uncontrolled muscle movements

Minor:
- constipation
- drowsiness
- dry mouth
- general feeling of discomfort or illness
- loss of appetite
- nervousness or restlessness
- difficulty sleeping

Time Required for Drug to Take Effect: Starts
to work within 30 to 60 minutes.

Symptoms of Overdose:
- cold, clammy skin
- severe confusion
- seizures

- severe dizziness or drowsiness
- continued nausea, vomiting, or diarrhea
- severe nervousness or restlessness
- difficulty breathing
- slowed heart beat

Special Notes:
- This medication may cause drowsiness. Do not operate a motor vehicle or other machinery while you are taking this medication.
- Morphine and other narcotics (such as oxycodone and codeine) cause constipation. This side effect may be diminished by drinking 6 to 8 full glasses of water each day. If using this medication for chronic pain, adding a stool softener–laxative combination may be necessary.
- Check with your physician or pharmacist before using any over-the-counter medications.
- When morphine is used over a long period of time, your body may become tolerant and require larger doses.
- Do not stop taking this medication abruptly.
- Nausea and vomiting may occur, especially after the first few doses. This effect may go away if you lie down for a while.
- If you experience dry mouth, try sugarless candy or gum, ice chips, or a saliva substitute.
- Do not drink alcohol while taking this medication.
- Sustained-release tablets should not be used for acute pain relief but to maintain a steady level of medication in the bloodstream for the treatment of chronic pain.

nabumetone

Brand Name: Relafen (SK Beecham)

Generic Available: no

Type of Drug: nonsteroidal anti-inflammatory drug (analgesic, anti-inflammatory, and antipyretic)

Used for: Treatment of pain associated with osteoarthritis or rheumatoid arthritis.

How This Medication Works: Inhibits substances called prostaglandins in the body that cause pain and inflammation.

Dosage Form and Strength: tablets (500 mg, 750 mg)

Storage:
- room temperature
- tightly closed
- protected from moisture and light

Administration:
- Usually taken 1 to 2 times daily.
- Take with meals or milk if stomach upset occurs.
- Take with a full glass of water (6 to 8 ounces).
- Do not lie down for at least 30 minutes after taking this medicine.

Precautions:
Do not use if:
- you are allergic to nabumetone or any other nonsteroidal anti-inflammatory drug such as ibuprofen, etodolac, indomethacin, piroxicam, or aspirin.

- medicine is beyond the expiration date or unusual in appearance.

Talk to your doctor if:

- you are taking aspirin; another nonsteroidal anti-inflammatory drug such as ibuprofen, etodolac, indomethacin, or piroxicam; anticoagulants such as warfarin; steroids such as prednisone; lithium; diuretics such as furosemide or hydrochloro-thiazide; methotrexate; or a beta blocker such as atenolol.
- you have peptic ulcer disease, bleeding from your stomach or intestines, bleeding abnormalities, ulcerative colitis, high blood pressure (hypertension), kidney disease, liver disease, heart disease, asthma, or nasal polyps.
- you smoke tobacco or drink alcohol.

Side Effects:

Major:

- blood in stool or dark, tarry stool
- persistent or severe stomach or abdominal pain
- vomiting blood
- blood in urine, or dark smokey-colored urine
- difficulty urinating
- rash
- difficulty breathing
- swelling of the eyelids, throat, lips, or face (allergic reaction)
- vision or hearing changes
- unexplained sore throat or fever
- unusual bleeding or bruising
- irregular heart beat
- yellowing of the skin or eyes (jaundice)

Minor:
- stomach upset
- gas or heartburn
- diarrhea or constipation
- swelling of hands or feet
- dizziness and drowsiness
- headache
- increased sensitivity to the sun or ultraviolet light

Time Required for Drug to Take Effect: Starts
to relieve pain in 1 to 2 hours. However, it may take
2 to 4 weeks to feel the full benefits of this medicine
when treating arthritis.

Symptoms of Overdose:
- stomach pain, nausea, or vomiting
- heartburn
- drowsiness
- headache
- confusion
- loss of consciousness

Special Notes:
- Alcohol may increase your risk of bleeding from
  the stomach or intestines while taking nabumetone.
- Contact physician if pain or fever worsens during
  self treatment.
- Use a sunblock with at least SPF 15 when outside
  because nabumetone may increase your sensitivity to the sun.
- Tell the doctor or dentist you are taking nabumetone if you are going to have surgery or emergency treatment.

naproxen
naproxen sodium

Brand Names:

Naproxen:
Naprosyn (Syntex)
Naprelan (Wyeth-Ayerst)

Naproxen sodium:
Anaprox (Syntex)
Aleve (Proctor & Gamble)

Generic Available: yes

Type of Drug: nonsteroidal anti-inflammatory drug (analgesic, anti-inflammatory, and antipyretic)

Used for: Treatment of pain associated with rheumatoid arthritis, osteoarthritis, gouty arthritis, headache, toothache, dental procedures, muscular aches, orthopedic procedures, backache, and injuries; can also be used to reduce a fever.

How This Medication Works: Inhibits substances called prostaglandins that cause pain and inflammation.

Dosage Form and Strength:

Naproxen:
- tablets (250 mg, 375 mg, 500 mg)
- delayed- or extended-release tablets (375 mg, 500 mg)
- oral suspension (125 mg/5 mL)

Naproxen sodium:
- tablets (220 mg [equivalent to naproxen 200 mg], 275 mg [equivalent to naproxen 250 mg], 550 mg [equivalent to naproxen 500 mg])

Storage:
- room temperature
- tightly closed
- protected from moisture and light

Administration:
- Usually taken 1 or 2 times daily.
- Adults taking nonprescription ibuprofen may take 200 to 400 mg every 8 to 12 hours, not to exceed 600 mg per 24-hour period.
- Take with meals or milk if stomach upset occurs.
- Take with a full glass of water (6 to 8 ounces).
- Shake suspension well before measuring dose.
- Do not lie down for at least 30 minutes after taking this medicine.
- Do not break, crush, or chew delayed- or extended-release tablets.

Precautions:
Do not use if:
- you are allergic to naproxen or any other non-steroidal anti-inflammatory drug such as ibu-profen, etodolac, piroxicam, or aspirin.
- medicine is beyond the expiration date or unusual in appearance.

Talk to your doctor if:
- you are taking aspirin, another nonsteroidal anti-inflammatory drug such as ibuprofen, etodolac, indomethacin, or piroxicam; anticoagulants such as warfarin; steroids such as prednisone; lithium; diuretics such as furosemide or hydrochloroth-iazide; methotrexate; or a beta blocker such as atenolol.

- you have peptic ulcer disease, bleeding from your stomach or intestines, bleeding abnormalities, ulcerative colitis, high blood pressure (hypertension), kidney disease, liver disease, heart disease, asthma, or nasal polyps.
- you smoke tobacco or drink alcohol.

Side Effects:

Major:

- blood in stool or dark, tarry stool
- persistent or severe stomach or abdominal pain
- vomiting blood
- blood in urine, dark smokey-colored urine
- difficulty urinating
- rash
- difficulty breathing
- swelling of the eyelids, throat, lips, or face
- vision or hearing changes
- unexplained sore throat or fever
- unusual bleeding or bruising

Minor:

- stomach upset or gas
- heartburn
- diarrhea or constipation
- swelling of hands or feet
- dizziness or drowsiness
- headache
- increased sensitivity to sun or ultraviolet light

Time Required for Drug to Take Effect: Starts to relieve pain in 1 to 2 hours. However, it may take 2 to 4 weeks to feel the full benefits of this medicine when treating arthritis.

Symptoms of Overdose:
- stomach pain, heartburn, nausea, and vomiting
- drowsiness
- headache
- seizures

Special Notes:
- Naproxen sodium may worsen heart failure, high blood pressure (hypertension), or ankle edema.
- Alcohol may increase your risk of bleeding from the stomach or intestines while taking naproxen.
- Self-medication with nonprescription naproxen should not exceed 10 days unless directed by a physician or pharmacist. Self-medication of fever should not exceed 3 days unless directed by a physician or pharmacist.
- Use a sunblock with at least SPF 15 when outside because naproxen may increase your sensitivity to the sun.
- Tell the doctor or dentist you are taking naproxen before undergoing any treatment.
- Contact physician if pain or fever worsens during self-treatment.

nefazodone

Brand Name: Serzone (Bristol-Myers Squibb)

Generic Available: no

Type of Drug: antidepressant

Used for: Treatment of depression.

How This Medication Works: Although it is not known exactly how nefazodone works, it appears to prolong the action of the neurotransmitters serotonin and norepinephrine and blocks the effect of serotonin in certain parts of the brain.

Dosage Form and Strength: tablets (100 mg, 150 mg, 200 mg, 250 mg)

Storage:
- room temperature
- tightly closed

Administration:
- Usually taken twice daily.

Precautions:
Do not use if:
- you are allergic to nefazodone or trazodone.
- you are taking astemizole or terfenadine.
- you are taking, or have taken in the past 14 days, a monoamine oxidase (MAO) inhibitor such as phenelzine or tranylcypromine.

Talk to your doctor if:
- you are taking alprazolam, triazolam, digoxin, propranolol, or haloperidol.
- you have ever had a stroke, heart disease, seizures, or liver problems.

Side Effects:
Major:
- dizziness or fainting when standing up
- clumsy or unsteady walking
- changes in vision
- unusual agitation, excitment, or confusion

- skin rash or itching
- ringing in the ears
- difficulty breathing
- severe nausea or vomiting
- difficulty urinating

Minor:
- dizziness, drowsiness, or confusion
- sleep problems or vivid dreams
- dry mouth
- constipation, diarrhea, or heartburn
- fever or chills
- headache
- tremor
- joint pain

Time Required for Drug to Take Effect: Full
benefit may take from 4 to 8 weeks to occur. Some
patients may notice improved appetite or sleep within
the first few weeks.

Symptoms of Overdose:
- nausea and vomiting
- severe drowsiness, dizziness, or confusion
- abnormal vision

Special Notes:
- Know which "target symptoms" (restlessness,
  worry, fear, or changes in sleep or appetite) you
  are being treated for and be prepared to tell your
  doctor if your target symptoms are improving,
  worsening, or unchanged.
- Do not discontinue without first talking with your
  doctor.
- Do not drink alcohol while taking this medication.

nicotine (topical)

Brand Names:

Habitrol (Basel)   Nicotrol (Parke-Davis)
Nicoderm (Marion   Prostep (Lederle)
  Merrell Dow)

Generic Available: no

Type of Drug: antismoking aid

Used for: Helping people to quit smoking.

How This Medication Works: Patches release
nicotine to prevent smoking withdrawal symptoms.

Dosage Form and Strength: patch
(5 mg/16 hours, 7 mg/24 hours, 10 mg/16 hours,
11 mg/24 hours, 14 mg/24 hours, 15 mg/16 hours,
21 mg/24 hours, 22 mg/24 hours)

Storage:
- room temperature
- in original packaging

Administration:
- Read directions for application and dosing
  closely because they vary among products.
- Wash and dry hands thoroughly before and after
  putting the patch on.
- Apply to a clean, dry, non-oily, and hairless area
  of the upper arms, chest, or stomach.
- Press the disk firmly in place with your palm for
  10 seconds, making sure there is good contact,
  especially around the edges.

- Do not put the patch on the exact same place each time; rotate patch placement so that you have at least 1 week in between repeating the patch in the same area.
- Do not apply on cuts or abrasions.
- Patches are applied once daily; follow directions for dosing from the manufacturer or your doctor.
- If you miss a dose, replace the patch as soon as you remember it. If it is time for the next dose, skip the missed dose; do not put on 2 patches.

Precautions:
Do not use if:
- you have had an allergic reaction to nicotine or any type of adhesive dressing or bandage.
- you have severe angina.
- you have had a recent heart attack.

Talk to your doctor if:
- you have mild angina, irregular heart rates, diabetes, high blood pressure (hypertension), hyperthyroidism, pheochromocytoma, stomach ulcer, or skin diseases.
- you have ever had a heart attack.
- you have not stopped smoking after 4 weeks.
- you are taking any other medication, especially theophylline, propranolol, or insulin.

Side Effects:
Major:
- nausea, vomiting, or diarrhea
- irregular heart beat
- stomach pain
- swelling

Minor:
- fast heart beat
- headache, mild
- increased appetite
- redness, burning, and itching at the patch site

Time Required for Drug to Take Effect:
Begins to enter the bloodstream immediately.

Symptoms of Overdose:
- confusion, seizures
- diarrhea, nausea, or stomach pain
- dilated pupils or eyes moving from side to side
- facial paralysis
- hearing loss or ringing in the ears (tinnitus)
- slowed breathing
- tingle of the arms and legs
- watery eyes and mouth

Special Notes:
- You must stop smoking when using the patches; nicotine overdoses can be fatal.
- Wash hands with water only; soap will increase absorption through the skin.
- To not take the patches by mouth; if accidentally taken orally, call your doctor or poison center.
- Do not use the patches more than 3 to 5 months.

nifedipine

Brand Names:

Adalat (Miles)

Adalat CC (Miles)

Procardia (Pfizer)

Procardia XL (Pfizer)

Generic Available: yes

Type of Drug: cardiovascular (calcium channel blocker)

Used for: Treatment of angina and high blood pressure (hypertension).

How This Medication Works: Inhibits smooth-muscle contraction and causes dilation in the blood carrying vessels in the body.

Dosage Form and Strength:
- sustained-release tablets (30 mg, 60 mg, 90 mg)
- capsules (10 mg, 20 mg)

Storage:
- room temperature
- protected from humidity

Administration:
- Swallow sustained-release tablets whole; do not crush or chew.
- Take at the same time every day.
- Adalat CC should be taken on an empty stomach.

Precautions:
Do not use if:
- you have ever had an allergic reaction to nifedipine or another calcium channel blocker such as amlodipine, diltiazem, or verapamil.

Talk to your doctor if:
- you have heart, kidney, or liver disease or problems with circulation or your blood vessels.
- you are taking any other medications, especially carbamazepine, cyclosporin, or warfarin.

Side Effects:

Major:
- bleeding or bruising, especially in the gum area
- skin rash, itching
- difficulty breathing
- painful or swollen joints, swollen legs
- chest pressure or discomfort
- fainting

Minor:
- light-headedness, dizziness, or drowsiness
- headache
- sexual dysfunction
- flushing
- nausea or constipation
- cough
- irritated gums

Time Required for Drug to Take Effect: Starts
to work within 20 minutes. However, it takes at least
2 to 4 weeks to see the maximal response.

Symptoms of Overdose:
- nausea and vomiting
- weakness, drowsiness, or slurred speech
- dizziness or confusion
- palpitations
- loss of consciousness

Special Notes:
- The short-acting forms of nifedipine should not be
  used to treat high blood pressure (hypertension).
- Nifedipine is used to prevent angina; sublingual
  capsules may be required to treat or relieve an
  acute attack of angina.

- Changing positions slowly when sitting and/or standing up may help decrease dizziness caused by this medication. If dizziness occurs, do not perform activities requiring mental alertness, such as driving a car or operating machinery.
- Check with your physician or pharmacist before using any over-the-counter medications.
- Avoid becoming dehydrated or overheated. Avoid saunas and exercise in hot weather; avoid alcoholic beverages; and drink plenty of fluids.
- The active drug in the extended-release tablets is released through osmosis. Sometimes the ghost of the tablet may show up in the stool and appear not to have been absorbed. However, the active ingredient will have been absorbed.

nitrofurantoin

Brand Names:

Macrodantin (Procter & Gamble)

Macrobid (Procter & Gamble)

Furadantin (Procter & Gamble)

Generic Available: yes

Type of Drug: anti-infective

Used for: Treatment of urinary tract infections.

How This Medication Works: Interferes with carbohydrate metabolism in the invading bacteria and disrupts bacterial cell wall formation.

Dosage Form and Strength:
- capsules (25 mg, 50 mg, 100 mg)
- suspension (25 mg/5 mL)

Storage:
- room temperature
- tightly closed
- protected from humidity

Administration:
- Take at even intervals.
- Take with food or milk to increase absorption and to decrease stomach upset.
- Take until completely gone, even if symptoms have improved.
- Shake suspension well before measuring dose.
- If using antacids, separate doses of nitrofurantoin and antacid by 2 hours.

Precautions:
Do not use if:
- you are allergic to nitrofurantoin.
- medicine is beyond the expiration date.

Talk to your doctor if:
- you are taking probenecid or magnesium supplements.
- you have ever had liver or kidney disease.

Side Effects:
Major:
- fever, chills, cough
- chest pain
- difficulty breathing
- skin rash

- numbness or tingling of the hands or feet
- persistent vomiting
- unexplained bruising
- confusion

Minor:
- brown discoloration of the urine
- nausea and vomiting
- abdominal pain
- headache
- dizziness and drowsiness

Time Required for Drug to Take Effect:
Begins to kill infecting bacteria within hours. However, you must continue to take nitrofurantoin for the full course of treatment, even if symptoms disappear.

Symptoms of Overdose:
- vomiting

Special Notes:
- Do not use for infections other than the one for which it was prescribed.

nitroglycerin

Brand Names:

Nitrostat (Parke-Davis)

Nitrolingual Spray
(Rhone-Poulenc Rorer)

Nitrong (Rhone-Poulenc
Rorer)

NitroBid Plateau caps
(Marion Merrell Dow)

Nitro-Dur (Key)

Transderm-Nitro (Summit)

Minitran (3M Pharm)

Nitrodisc (Roberts)

Nitrol Oint (Savage)

Nitro-Bid Oint (Marion
Merrell Dow)

Generic Available:
- sublingual tablets: yes
- sublingual spray: no
- spray ointment: yes
- skin patches: no
- sustained-release capsules: yes
- sustained-release tablets: no

Type of Drug: antianginal

Used for: Treatment of chest pain, congestive heart failure, angina, and coronary heart disease.

How This Medication Works: Relaxes smooth muscle, reducing blood pressure and demand on heart.

Dosage Form and Strength:
- sublingual tablets (0.3 mg, 0.4 mg, 0.6 mg)
- sustained-release capsules (2.5 mg, 2.6 mg, 6.5 mg, 9 mg, 13 mg)
- sublingual spray (0.4 mg per spray)
- ointment (1 inch contains 15 mg)
- skin patches (0.1 mg/hr, 0.2 mg/hr, 0.3 mg/hr, 0.4 mg/hr, 0.6 mg/hr, 0.8 mg/hr)

Storage:
- room temperature
- tightly closed in original container
- protected from humidity

Administration:
- Oral or sustained-release products are usually taken twice daily.
- Sublingual tablets (or the spray) are taken when necessary to relieve chest pain.

- If you experience chest pain, place 1 sublingual tablet or spray under the tongue and let it dissolve; do not swallow. If pain persists after 5 minutes, take another dose. Repeat again in 5 minutes, if needed. If pain is not relieved after 3 doses, seek immediate medical attention.
- It is important to have an 8- to 10-hour period each day that is drug free. If nitrates (such as nitroglycerin and isosorbide) are taken continuously, tolerance will develop and the medication becomes ineffective. Skin patches should be removed for at least 8 hours daily. The ointment should be applied every 6 hours, but only 3 times daily (for example, 8 A.M., 2 P.M., and 8 P.M.). Capsules should be taken 8 hours apart, but only 2 times a day (for example, 8 A.M., and 4 P.M.).
- Take on an empty stomach, 1 hour before or 2 hours after a meal.
- Dissolve sublingual tablets under the tongue, do not swallow, crush, or chew.
- Use sublingual products only when seated.
- Ointment should be applied to the chest or back using the applicator or dose-measuring paper not your fingers; spread the ointment in a uniform layer over an area that is roughly the size of the applicator paper.
- Do not rub or massage the ointment.
- Patches should be applied to the chest, upper back, or upper arms. Apply to an area that has no cuts, is free of hair, and is not irritated. Try to avoid areas that will be subject to the movement of your arms.

- If using skin patches, and you predictably experience chest pain with activity, wear the patch during the day and take it off at night. If you experience night time shortness of breath or chest pain at night or in the early morning, wear the patch at night and take it off for 8 hours during the day.
- Sublingual spray or tablets may be used 5 or 10 minutes before an activity that might cause chest pain.

Precautions:
Do not use if:
- you are allergic to nitroglycerin or other medicines in the nitrate family such as isosorbide mononitrate or isosorbide dinitrate.
- medicine is beyond the expiration date.

Talk to your doctor if:
- you have glaucoma or severe anemia.
- you are taking a calcium channel blocker such as nifedipine, amlodipine, diltiazem, or verapamil.
- you have allergies to adhesives and the doctor has prescribed the topical patch.

Side Effects:
Major:
- fainting
- chest pain
- blurred vision
- dry mouth

Minor:
- headache
- dizziness, flushing, or weakness
- nausea, diarrhea, or stomach upset

Time Required for Drug to Take Effect:
Sublingual tablets and spray begins to work in 2 to
5 minutes; the ointment begins to work in about
30 minutes and continues to have an effect for 4 to
6 hours. Sustained-release capsule begins to work in
about 4 hours and continues to work for up to 8 hours.

Symptoms of Overdose:
- very low blood pressure (fainting)
- rapid heart beat
- visual disturbances
- shortness of breath

Special Notes:
- Changing positions slowly when sitting and/or
  standing up may help decrease dizziness caused
  by this medication.
- If you notice dizziness, avoid activities requiring
  mental alertness, such as operating a motor
  vehicle or dangerous machinery.
- Do not drink alcohol while taking this medication.
- Do not change brands of this drug without consulting your pharmacist or physician.
- Use sublingual products for acute angina attacks.
- Do not use oral capsules or transdermal patches
  for acute angina attacks.
- There will still be some nitroglycerin left in the
  patch after you remove it. Discard it carefully,
  being mindful of the safety of children and pets.
- Do not inhale spray.
- A sublingual tablet that does not burn or sting
  will still be effective.

nizatidine

Brand Name: Axid Pulvules (Lilly)

Generic Available: no

Type of Drug: Gastrointestinal (histamine H_2 antagonist)

Used for: Treatment of excess acid production in the stomach, ulcers, and heartburn (gastroesophageal reflux disease [GERD]).

How This Medication Works: Blocks the binding of histamine to sites that would cause acid secretion.

Dosage Form and Strength: capsules (150 mg, 300 mg)

Storage:
- room temperature
- protected from humidity

Administration:
- If you are taking multiple doses daily, take with or immediately after meals, unless your doctor has different instructions.
- If you are only taking 1 dose per day, take it before bedtime, unless directed otherwise.
- If using antacids, separate doses of nizatidine and antacid by 2 hours.

Precautions:

Do not use if:
- you are allergic to nizatidine or other histamine H_2 antagonists such as cimetidine or ranitidine.

Talk to your doctor if:
- you have kidney or liver disease.
- you are taking any other medications, especially theophylline, anticoagulants (such as warfarin), antidepressants (such as amitriptyline, fluoxetine, or trazodone), antibiotics, phenytoin, and medications for heart disease or high blood pressure.

Side Effects:
Major:
- skin rash, hives, or itching
- blurred vision or confusion
- irregular heartbeat or tightness in chest
- fever and sore throat
- swelling of eyelids
- unusual bleeding or bruising

Minor:
- constipation or diarrhea
- decreased sexual ability or desire
- dizziness or drowsiness
- headache
- dry mouth
- increased sweating
- joint or muscle pain
- loss of appetite
- nausea or vomiting
- ringing or buzzing in the ears (tinnitus)
- swelling of breasts (in men and women)
- hair loss

Time Required for Drug to Take Effect: Starts
to work within 1 to 2 hours, but ulcer healing may require 4 to 12 weeks of therapy.

Symptoms of Overdose:
- difficulty breathing
- irregular heartbeat
- tremors
- vomiting
- diarrhea
- light-headedness

Special Notes:
- Check with your physician or pharmacist before using any over-the-counter medications.
- Avoid medications that may make your ulcer worse, including nonsteroidal anti-inflammatory drugs (such as aspirin, ibuprofen, naproxen, and ketoprofen).
- If you are smoking, you should quit. If you continue to smoke, you should try not to smoke after the last dose of nizatidine for the day.
- This medication may cause drowsiness. Use caution when operating a motor vehicle or operating dangerous machinery.
- Avoid alcohol or other medications that may make you drowsy or dizzy, such as antihistamines, sedatives, tranquilizers, sleeping medications, pain relievers, seizure medications, and muscle relaxants.
- Tell the doctor you are taking nizatidine if you are going to have a skin test for allergies.
- If you experience dryness of the mouth, try sugarless candy or gum, ice chips, or a saliva substitute.
- Tell the doctor or dentist you are taking nizatidine if you are going to have surgery or emergency treatment.

nortriptyline

Brand Names:
Aventyl (Lilly)
Pamelor (Sandoz)

Generic Available: yes

Type of Drug: tricyclic antidepressant

Used for: Treatment of depression, chronic pain, and panic disorder.

How This Medication Works: Increases the action of the neurotransmitters norepinephrine and serotonin.

Dosage Form and Strength:
- capsules (10 mg, 25 mg, 50 mg, 75 mg)
- liquid/solution (10 mg/5 cc)

Storage:
- room temperature
- tightly closed

Administration:
- Usually taken once daily at bedtime; may also be prescribed 2 to 3 times daily.
- May be taken without regard to food.
- Liquid medicine should be measured using an accurate measure (available in pharmacies).

Precautions:
Do not use if:
- you are allergic to nortriptyline or another tricyclic antidepressant such as amitriptyline.

- you are also taking a monoamine oxidase (MAO) inhibitor such as phenelzine or selegiline.

Talk to your doctor if:

- you have glaucoma (angle closure type), heart disease, urinary or prostate problems, severe constipation, breathing problems, seizures, diabetes, or a thyroid problem.
- you are taking cimetidine, clonidine, methyldopa, reserpine, guanethidine, sedatives, muscle relaxants, antihistamines, decongestants (including cold medications), or stimulants.
- you drink alcohol.

Side Effects:

Major:

- dizziness or fainting
- rapid heart beat
- chest pain
- confusion or hallucinations
- severe constipation or urinary retention
- rash
- severe sedation
- fever
- restlessness or agitation
- severe sunburn

Minor:

- drowsiness
- dry mouth
- mild constipation
- weight gain
- unpleasant taste
- stomach upset

Time Required for Drug to Take Effect: May take from 4 to 8 weeks for full antidepressant benefit; improvement may occur within 1 to 2 weeks for certain symptoms.

Symptoms of Overdose:
- confusion or hallucinations
- seizures
- extreme sedation
- very slow or rapid heart beat
- difficulty breathing
- inability to urinate
- severe constipation
- dilated pupils

Special Notes:
- Know which "target symptoms" (restlessness, worry, fear, or changes in sleep or appetite) you are being treated for and be prepared to tell your doctor if your target symptoms are improving, worsening, or unchanged.
- Nortriptyline can be measured in the blood. Your doctor may order a blood test to determine the level of nortrityline in your body.
- Do not discontinue and never increase your dose without the advice of your doctor.
- Check with your physician or pharmacist before using any over-the-counter medications.
- If you have diabetes, you may need to check your blood glucose more frequently.
- Use a sunblock with at least SPF 15 when outside because nortriptyline may increase your sensitivity to the sun.

olsalazine

Brand Name: Dipentum (Pharmacia)

Generic Available: no

Type of Drug: gastrointestinal

Used for: Treatment of ulcerative colitis.

How This Medication Works: Decreases the inflammation in the bowel to reduce symptoms.

Dosage Form and Strength: capsules (250 mg)

Storage:
- room temperature
- protected from humidity

Administration:
- Take olsalazine with food to decrease stomach upset and diarrhea.

Precautions:
Do not use if:
- you are allergic to olsalazine, aspirin, mesalamine, sulfasalazine, or salicylates.

Talk to your doctor if:
- you have kidney disease.
- you are taking any other medications.

Side Effects:
Major:
- skin rash, hives, or itching
- bloody diarrhea
- fever, sore throat

- pale skin
- unusual bleeding or bruising
- yellow eyes or skin (jaundice)

Minor:
- abdominal pain, stomach upset, or diarrhea
- nausea or vomiting
- acne
- drowsiness
- difficulty sleeping
- muscle or joint aches

Time Required for Drug to Take Effect: Starts to work as soon as it reaches the intestines.

Symptoms of Overdose:
- decreased ability to move
- diarrhea

Special Notes:
- Check with your physician or pharmacist before using any over-the-counter medications.

omeprazole

Brand Name: Prilosec (Merck)

Generic Available: no

Type of Drug: gastrointestinal (proton pump inhibitor)

Used for: Treatment of excess acid production in the stomach, ulcers, and heartburn (gastroesophageal reflux disease [GERD]).

How This Medication Works: Inhibits the mechanism that transports acid into the stomach.

Dosage Form and Strength: sustained-release capsules (20 mg)

Storage:
- room temperature
- protected from humidity

Administration:
- Take immediately before a meal, preferably in the morning.
- Swallow the capsule whole. Do not crush, chew, break, or open.

Precautions:
Do not use if:
- you are allergic to omeprazole or lansoprazole.

Talk to your doctor if:
- you have liver disease.
- you are taking any other medications, especially diazepam, phenytoin, and anticoagulants such as warfarin.

Side Effects:
Major:
- skin rash, hives, or itching
- ulcers or sores in mouth
- difficult or frequent urination
- fever or sore throat
- unusual bleeding or bruising

Minor:
- stomach discomfort
- constipation or diarrhea

- gas or heartburn
- headache
- muscle pain
- nausea and vomiting
- drowsiness or dizziness

Time Required for Drug to Take Effect:
Begins to work in several days.

Symptoms of Overdose:
- cold temperature
- drowsiness
- seizures or convulsions
- difficulty breathing

Special Notes:
- Check with your physician or pharmacist before using any over-the-counter medications.
- Avoid medications that may make your ulcer worse, including nonsteroidal anti-inflammatory drugs (such as aspirin, ibuprofen, and naproxen).
- If you smoke, you should quit. If you continue to smoke, you should try not to smoke after the last dose of omeprazole for the day.
- Do not drink alcohol while taking this medication.

oxaprozin

Brand Name: Daypro (Searle)

Generic Available: no

Type of Drug: nonsteroidal anti-inflammatory drug (analgesic, anti-inflammatory, and antipyretic)

Used for: Treatment of relief of pain in osteoarthritis and rheumatoid arthritis.

How This Medication Works: Inhibits substances called prostaglandins that cause pain and inflammation.

Dosage Form and Strength: tablets (600 mg)

Storage:
- room temperature
- tightly closed
- protected from moisture and sunlight

Administration:
- Usually taken once daily.
- Take with meals or milk if stomach upset occurs.
- Do not lie down for at least 30 minutes after taking this medicine.
- Take with a full glass of water (6 to 8 ounces).

Precautions:

Do not use if:
- you are allergic to oxaprozin or any other non-steroidal anti-inflammatory drug such as ibuprofen, etodolac, indomethacin, piroxicam, or aspirin.
- medicine is beyond the expiration date or unusual in appearance.

Talk to your doctor if:
- you are taking aspirin; another nonsteroidal anti-inflammatory drug such as ibuprofen, etodolac, or piroxicam; anticoagulants such as warfarin; steroids such as prednisone; lithium; diuretics such as furosemide or hydrochlorothiazide; methotrexate; or a beta blocker such as atenolol.

- you have peptic ulcer disease, bleeding from your stomach or intestines, bleeding abnormalities, ulcerative colitis, high blood pressure (hypertension), kidney disease, liver disease, heart disease, asthma, anemia, or nasal polyps.
- you smoke tobacco or drink alcohol.

Side Effects:

Major:
- blood in stool or dark, tarry stool
- persistent or severe stomach or abdominal pain
- vomiting blood
- blood in urine, dark smokey-colored urine
- difficulty urinating
- rash
- difficulty breathing
- swelling of the eyelids, throat, lips, or face
- vision or hearing changes
- unexplained sore throat or fever
- unusual bleeding or bruising
- irregular heart beat

Minor:
- stomach upset or gas
- heartburn
- diarrhea or constipation
- swelling of hands or feet
- dizziness or drowsiness
- headache
- increased sensitivity to the sun or ultraviolet light

Time Required for Drug to Take Effect: It may take 2 to 4 weeks to feel the full benefits when treating arthritis.

Symptoms of Overdose:
- stomach pain or heartburn
- nausea and vomiting
- drowsiness, confusion, or loss of consciousness
- headache

Special Notes:
- Drinking alcohol or smoking tobacco may increase your risk of bleeding from the stomach or intestines while taking oxaprozin.
- Use a sunblock with at least SPF 15 when outside because oxaprozin may increase your sensitivity to the sun.
- Tell the doctor or dentist you are taking oxaprozin before undergoing any treatment.
- Contact physician if pain worsens during treatment.

oxazepam

Brand Name: Serax (Wyeth-Ayerst)

Generic Available: yes

Type of Drug: antianxiety

Used for: Treatment of anxiety.

How This Medication Works: Enhances the neurotransmitter gamma amino butyric acid to depress the central nervous system and reduce anxiety.

Dosage Form and Strength:
- tablets (15 mg)
- capsules (10 mg, 15 mg, 30 mg)

Storage:
- room temperature
- tightly closed

Administration:
- Usually taken 3 to 4 times daily.
- Take with food if stomach upset occurs.

Precautions:
Do not use if:
- you have ever had an allergic reaction to oxazepam or other drugs in the benzodiazepine family such as diazepam, lorazepam, or triazolam.

Talk to your doctor if:
- you are taking any other medications, especially those that may depress the central nervous system such as alcohol, phenobarbital, or narcotics (such as codeine, meperidine, or morphine).
- you have asthma or other lung problems, kidney disease, or liver disease.
- you have been told that you snore.

Side Effects:
Major:
- difficulty concentrating or confusion
- seizures
- hallucinations
- rash

Minor:
- unsteadiness, drowsiness, or slurred speech
- blurred vision

Time Required for Drug to Take Effect:
Begins to lessen anxiety within 2 hours of taking a dose.

Symptoms of Overdose:
- continuing confusion or slurred speech
- severe weakness or drowsiness
- shortness of breath

Special Notes:
- This medication may cause drowsiness. Use caution when operating a motor vehicle or operating dangerous machinery.
- Do not drink alcohol while taking this medication.
- Do not discontinue without first talking with your doctor.

oxybutynin

Brand Name: Ditropan (Marion Merrell Dow)

Generic Available: yes

Type of Drug: urinary tract stimulant

Used for: Treatment of urge incontinence and neurogenic bladder.

How This Medication Works: Decreases spasms in the bladder.

Dosage Form and Strength:
- tablets 5 mg
- syrup 5 mg/5 mL

Storage:
- room temperature
- tightly closed
- protected from light

Administration:
- Usually 5 mg 2 to 4 times daily.
- Take with food or milk to reduce stomach upset.
- If you miss a dose, take it as soon as you remember it, unless it is almost time for the next dose; do not double the dose.

Precautions:
Do not use if:
- you have had an allergic reaction to oxybutynin.

Talk to your doctor if:
- you have heart disease (mitral stenosis, irregular rhythms, congestive heart failure, coronary heart disease), gastrointestinal obstruction, glaucoma, hiatal hernia or reflux disease, paralytic ileus, myasthenia gravis, prostate enlargement, ulcerative colitis, or urinary retention.
- you are taking any other medication, especially anticholinergic agents such as certain antidepressants, antipsychotics, antihistamine, anti-Parkinson agents, and antispasmodics.

Side Effects:
Major:
- agitation, nervousness, or restlessness
- breathing difficulty
- fever
- flushing
- hallucinations
- increased heart rate

Minor:
- constipation
- drowsiness

- dry mouth, nose, and throat
- impotence
- nausea and vomiting
- sleeping difficulty
- decreased sweating
- vision changes (blurred vision or light sensitivity)

Time Required for Drug to Take Effect: May
take up to a few months to reach maximal effectiveness.

Symptoms of Overdose:
- agitation
- breathing difficulty
- confusion, disorientation, or hallucinations
- severe drowsiness
- fever
- irregular heart beat (fast or slow)
- pupil enlargement
- seizures
- vomiting
- weakness

Special Notes:
- Do not take while you have a fever because it may increase your temperature.
- Dentures may not fit as well or may irritate gums because oxybutynin often causes dry mouth.
- Do not drink alcohol while taking this medication.
- This medication may cause drowsiness. Use caution when operating a motor vehicle or dangerous machinery.
- If you experience dryness of the mouth, try sugarless candy or gum, ice chips, or a saliva substitute.

- Oxybutynin decreases your body's ability to sweat. Be careful to avoid getting overheated by outdoor activities in the heat, saunas, or hot baths and showers.

oxycodone
oxycodone and acetminophen combination

Brand Names:
Percocet (DuPont)
Roxicet (Roxane)
Tylox (McNeil)

OxyContin (Purdue-Frederick)
Roxicodone (Roxane)

Generic Available: yes

Type of Drug: analgesic

Used for: Relief of moderate to severe pain, suppression of cough, and treatment of diarrhea.

How This Medication Works: Oxycodone acts in the central nervous system to decrease the recognition of pain impulses. Acetaminophen works in the peripheral nervous system and blocks pain impulses.

Dosage Form and Strength:
Oxycodone and acetaminophen combination:
- tablets (5 mg oxycodone//325 mg acetaminophen)
- capsules (5 mg/500 mg)
- caplet (5 mg/500 mg)
- liquid (5 mg/325 mg per 5 mL)

Oxycodone:
- tablets (5 mg)
- sustained-release tablets (10 mg, 20 mg, 40 mg)
- liquid (5 mg/5 mL, 20 mg/mL)

Storage:
- room temperature
- protected from humidity

Administration:
- The tablets, capsules, and solution are usually taken every 4 hours.
- Sustained-release tablets are usually taken every 12 hours.
- The amount of oxycodone per dose is individualized for each patient and depends on the pain being treated and previous exposure to oxycodone.
- Each agent can be harmful if used in excess. Never take more tablets per dose or more doses per day than your doctor has prescribed.
- Take with milk or food if stomach upset occurs.
- Do not crush or chew sustained-release tablet.

Precautions:
Do not use if:
- you are allergic to oxycodone or other narcotics such as morphine, hydrocodone, hydromorphone, or codeine.
- you are allergic to acetaminophen.

Talk to your doctor if:
- you have alcoholism or other substance abuse problems; brain disease or head injury; colitis; seizures; emotional problems or mental illness; emphysema, asthma, or other lung diseases;

kidney, liver, or thyroid disease; prostate problems or problems with urination; or gallbladder disease or gallstones.

- you are taking naltrexone, zidovudine, or any other medications, especially those that can cause drowsiness such as antihistamines, barbiturates (phenobarbital), benzodiazepines (such as diazepam, alprazolam, and lorazepam), muscle relaxants, or antidepressants.

Side Effects:

Major:
- skin rash or hives
- irregular breathing or difficulty breathing
- fainting
- severe confusion or hallucinations
- painful, difficult, or frequent urination
- fast, slow, or pounding heart beat
- depression
- unusual bruising or bleeding
- trembling or uncontrolled muscle movements
- yellow eyes or skin (jaundice)

Minor:
- constipation
- drowsiness
- dry mouth
- general feeling of discomfort or illness
- loss of appetite
- nervousness, restlessness, or difficulty sleeping

Time Required for Drug to Take Effect: Starts
to work within 10 to 30 minutes. The sustained-release tablets begin to work within 1 hour.

Symptoms of Overdose:

- cold, clammy skin
- seizures
- severe dizziness, drowsiness, or confusion
- continued nausea, vomiting, or diarrhea
- severe nervousness or restlessness
- difficulty breathing
- slowed heart beat

(Symptoms associated with acetaminophen may not occur until 2 to 4 days after the overdose is taken, but it is important to begin treatment as soon as possible to prevent liver damage or death.)

Special Notes:

- This medication may cause drowsiness. Do not operate a motor vehicle or other machinery while you are taking this medication.
- Oxycodone and other narcotics cause constipation. This side effect may be diminished by drinking 6 to 8 full glasses of water each day. If using this medication for chronic pain, adding a stool softener–laxative combination may be necessary.
- Check with your physician or pharmacist before using any over-the-counter medications.
- When oxycodone is used for a long period, you may become tolerant and require larger doses.
- Do not stop taking this medication abruptly.
- Nausea and vomiting may occur, especially after the first few doses. This effect may go away if you lie down for a while.
- If you experience dryness of the mouth, try sugarless candy or gum, ice chips, or a saliva substitute.
- Do not drink alcohol while taking this medication.

- Sustained-release tablets should not be used for acute pain but for the treatment of chronic pain.
- If you think you or anyone else may have taken an overdose, get emergency help immediately.

paroxetine

Brand Name: Paxil (SK Beecham)

Generic Available: no

Type of Drug: antidepressant (selective serotonin reuptake inhibitor)

Used for: Treatment of depression.

How This Medication Works: Prolongs the effects of the neurotransmitter serotonin by interfering with its reuptake into nerve cells in the brain.

Dosage Form and Strength: tablets (20 mg, 30 mg)

Storage:
- room temperature
- tightly closed

Administration:
- Usually taken once daily in the morning or at bedtime (if you experience drowsiness).

Precautions:
Do not use if:
- you are allergic to paroxetine or other selective serotonin reuptake inhibitor antidepressants such as fluvoxamine or sertraline.

- you are currently taking, or have taken in the last 14 days, a monoamine oxidase (MAO) inhibitor such as phenelzine or tranylcypromine.

Talk to your doctor if:
- you have ever had liver problems, kidney problems, or seizures.
- you are taking phenobarbital, phenytoin, cimetidine, digoxin, procyclidine, a blood thinner (such as warfarin), or tryptophan.

Side Effects:

Major:
- seizures
- unusual agitation or restless
- dizziness, light-headedness, or fainting
- severe nausea or vomiting
- chest pain or palpitations

Minor:
- dizziness or drowsiness
- vivid dreams or insomnia
- headache
- tremor
- nausea
- decreased appetite, weight loss
- increased appetite, weight gain
- constipation
- decreased sexual function and desire
- tingling in hands and feet
- unusually strong reflex reactions

Time Required for Drug to Take Effect: May start to improve some symptoms within the first few weeks, but the full benefit may take from 4 to 8 weeks.

Symptoms of Overdose:

- seizures
- severe drowsiness
- dilated pupils
- very rapid heartbeat
- severe nausea or vomiting

Special Notes:

- Know which "target symptoms" (restlessness, worry, fear, or changes in sleep or appetite) you are being treated for and be prepared to tell your doctor if your target symptoms are improving, worsening, or unchanged.
- Paroxetine may interact with several other medicines commonly used by older adults. Show your doctor and pharmacist a complete list of all medicines, including nonprescription medicines.
- Do not drink alcohol while taking this medication.
- Never increase your dose without the advice of your doctor.

pentazocine

Brand Name: Talwin (Sanofi Winthrop)

Generic Available: no

Type of Drug: analgesic

Used for: Relief of pain.

How This Medication Works: Decreases the recognition of pain impulses in the central nervous system.

Dosage Form and Strength: tablets (50 mg)

Storage:
- room temperature
- protected from humidity

Administration:
- Do not exceed the maximum number of doses per day; never take more tablets per dose than your doctor has prescribed.
- Take with food or milk if stomach upset occurs.

Precautions:
Do not use if:
- you are allergic to pentazocine.

Talk to your doctor if:
- you have alcoholism or other substance abuse problems; brain disease or head injury; colitis; seizures; emotional problems or mental illness; emphysema, asthma, or other lung diseases; kidney, liver, or thyroid disease; prostate problems or problems with urination; or gallbladder disease or gallstones.
- you are taking naltrexone, zidovudine, or any other medications, especially those that can cause drowsiness such as antihistamines, barbiturates (phenobarbital), benzodiazepines (diazepam, lorazepam), muscle relaxants, or antidepressants.

Side Effects:
Major:
- skin rash or hives
- severe confusion or hallucinations
- irregular breathing or difficulty breathing

- painful, difficult, or frequent urination
- fast, slow, or pounding heartbeat
- depression
- trembling or uncontrolled muscle movements

Minor:
- constipation
- drowsiness
- dry mouth
- general feeling of discomfort or illness
- loss of appetite
- nervousness, restlessness, or difficulty sleeping

Time Required for Drug to Take Effect: Starts to work within 30 to 60 minutes.

Symptoms of Overdose:
- cold, clammy skin
- seizures
- severe dizziness, drowsiness, or confusion
- continued nausea, vomiting, or diarrhea
- severe nervousness or restlessness
- difficulty breathing
- slowed heartbeat

Special Notes:
- This medication may cause drowsiness. Do not operate a motor vehicle or other machinery.
- Pentazocine may cause constipation. This side effect may be diminished by drinking 6 to 8 full glasses of water each day. If using this medication for chronic pain, adding a stool softener–laxative combination may be necessary.
- Check with your physician or pharmacist before using any over-the-counter medications.

- When pentazocine is used over a long period of time, your body may become tolerant and require larger doses.
- Do not stop taking this medication abruptly.
- Nausea and vomiting may occur after the first few doses but may go away if you lie down.
- If you experience dryness of the mouth, try sugarless candy or gum, ice chips, or a saliva substitute.
- Do not drink alcohol while taking this medication.
- Sustained-release tablets should not be used for acute pain but for the treatment of chronic pain.
- If you think you or anyone else may have taken an overdose, get emergency help immediately.

pergolide

Brand Name: Permax (Lilly)

Generic Available: no

Type of Drug: antiparkinsonian

Used for: Treatment of Parkinson disease.

How This Medication Works: Mimics the action of the neurotransmitter dopamine, which is lacking in Parkinson disease.

Dosage Form and Strength: tablets (0.05 mg, 0.25 mg, 1 mg)

Storage:
- room temperature
- tightly closed

Administration:
- Usually administered 3 times daily with meals.
- Very low doses are used at first, then slowly increased over days and weeks to the full dose.
- Dosing schedules are individualized to prevent unpleasant side effects.

Precautions:
Do not use if:
- you have had an allergic reaction to pergolide or other ergot alkaloids such as bromocriptine.

Talk to your doctor if:
- you have heart disease.
- you get light-headed or dizzy after you sit up or stand up.
- you are taking metoclopramide or antipsychotic medications such as haloperidol or thioridazine.

Side Effects:
Major:
- seizures
- unusual decrease in blood pressure
- fainting
- agitation
- hallucinations
- severe nausea or vomiting

Minor:
- stomach upset
- dizziness or light-headedness when sitting up or standing up
- drowsiness
- insomnia
- nightmares

- constipation
- diarrhea
- stuffy nose
- dry mouth

Time Required for Drug to Take Effect: May
take weeks to months for maximum benefit (because
pergolide doses must be increased very slowly to avoid
serious side effects).

Symptoms of Overdose:
- seizures
- severe vomiting
- fainting
- unusually low blood pressure
- extreme agitation
- hallucinations

Special Notes:
- Pergolide may be used alone in early (mild)
  Parkinson disease, or it may be added to other
  medications when treating more advanced
  Parkinson disease. When it is added to other medications, your doctor may adjust the doses of
  other medications as you begin to respond.
- Your medication regimen may become more
  complicated. If you are having difficulty keeping
  track of your medication schedule, talk with your
  doctor or pharmacist. Skipping doses or accidentally taking extra doses can be dangerous.
- Patients who have some confusion or emotional
  or memory problems may be more sensitive to
  this medicine. If you notice any changes in
  behavior or emotions, talk with your doctor.

perphenazine

Brand Name: Trilafon (Schering)

Generic Available: yes

Type of Drug: antipsychotic

Used for: Treatment of psychotic disorders, nausea, and vomiting.

How This Medication Works: Blocks neurotransmitters in the central nervous system.

Dosage Form and Strength:
- tablets (2 mg, 4 mg, 8 mg, 16 mg)
- oral solution (16 mg/5 mL)

Storage:
- room temperature
- tightly closed

Administration:
- Usually taken 2 to 4 times daily.
- Oral solution may be diluted in a beverage such as water or juice (except apple juice).
- Do not mix oral solution with caffeinated beverages.
- Take with food or milk if stomach upset occurs.

Precautions:
Do not use if:
- you have had an allergic reaction to perphenazine or other medications from the phenothiazine family such as chlorpromazine or thioridazine.
- you have Parkinson disease.

Talk to your doctor if:
- you are taking any other medications, especially antacids, antidiarrheals, phenobarbital, carbamazepine, lithium, meperidine, propranolol, and tricyclic antidepressants (such as amitriptyline).
- you have liver disease, stomach ulcers, seizures, heart disease, or enlarged prostate.

Side Effects:
Major:
- blurred vision
- skin rash or sunburn
- problems speaking or swallowing
- lip smacking
- restlessness

Minor:
- constipation
- dizziness or drowsiness
- dry mouth

Time Required for Drug to Take Effect: Takes
several weeks before desired effect is seen.

Symptoms of Overdose:
- extreme drowsiness
- agitation, restlessness, or seizures
- fever

Special Notes:
- Do not drink alcohol while taking this medication.
- Do not discontinue without your doctor's consent.
- Tell your doctor about any involuntary muscle movements or spasms.
- Do not allow solution to touch skin.

phenazopyridine

Brand Name: Pyridium (Parke-Davis)

Generic Available: yes

Type of Drug: urinary tract analgesic

Used for: Prevention of painful urination.

How This Medication Works: Mechanism is unknown.

Dosage Form and Strength: tablets (100 mg, 200 mg)

Storage:
- room temperature
- tightly closed
- protected from light

Administration:
- Usually 200 mg 3 times daily for 3 to 15 days.
- Take after meals.

Precautions:
Do not use if:
- you are allergic to phenazopyridine.
- you have kidney or liver disease.

Talk to your doctor if:
- you are taking any other medication.

Side Effects:
Major:
- anemia or yellowing of the skin or eyes (jaundice)
- skin rash or itching

Minor:
- dizziness or headache
- red or orange urine
- stomach upset

Time Required for Drug to Take Effect: Starts to work in 1 to 2 days.

Symptoms of Overdose:
- anemia
- deeply stained urine or vomitus
- liver or kidney failure
- yellow skin pigmentation or eyes (jaundice)

Special Notes:
- Phenazopyridine is not an antibiotic and will not cure a urinary tract infection.
- Phenazopyridine can cause incorrect readings on urinalysis laboratory tests and home urinary glucose and ketone tests.
- Phenazopyridine should not be used long term.
- Urine may turn red or orange; if clothing or bedding is stained, try soaking in a 0.25% solution of sodium dithionite or sodium hydrosulfite.

phenobarbital

Brand Name: none

Generic Available: yes

Type of Drug: anticonvulsant

Used for: Treatment of epilepsy.

How This Medication Works: Depresses central
nervous system to prevent seizures.

Dosage Form and Strength:
- tablets (15 mg, 30 mg, 60 mg, 100 mg)
- oral elixir (15 mg/5 mL, 20 mg/5 mL)

Storage:
- room temperature
- tightly closed container

Administration:
- Usually taken 2 to 3 times daily.
- Take tablets whole; do not crush or chew.

Precautions:
Do not use if:
- you are allergic to phenobarbital or any other
  medications in the barbiturate family.

Talk to your doctor if:
- you are taking any other medication, especially
  rifampin, valproic acid, warfarin, beta blockers
  (specifically propranolol and metoprolol), carbamazepine, clonazepam, corticosteroids such as
  prednisone, doxycycline, felodipine, phenytoin,
  quinidine, theophylline, verapamil, and monamine oxidase (MAO) inhibitors such as phenelzine and tranylcypromine.
- you have liver disease, kidney disease, diabetes,
  asthma, or anemia.

Side Effects:
Major:
- confusion
- hallucinations

Minor:
- clumsiness
- dizziness
- light-headedness
- constipation
- nausea and vomiting

Time Required for Drug to Take Effect:

Therapy with this medication decreases the number and/or frequency of seizures as long as the medication is continued.

Symptoms of Overdose:

- severe or continuing confusion
- irritability
- weakness
- slurred speech
- shortness of breath

Special Notes:

- This medication may cause drowsiness. Use caution when operating a motor vehicle or dangerous machinery.
- Check with your physician or pharmacist before using any other medication, including over-the-counter medications.
- Do not drink alcohol while taking this medication.
- Do not discontinue without first talking with your doctor or pharmacist.
- You will occasionally have blood drawn to monitor the amount of phenobarbital in your blood.

phenylpropanolamine and chlorpheniramine combination

Brand Names:

Condrin-LA (Hauck)
Contac 12-Hour (SK Beecham)
Drize (Ascher)
Dura-Vent/A (Dura)
Oragest T.D. (Major)

Ornade (SK Beecham)
Resaid S.R. (Geneva)
Rhinolar-Ex (McGregor)
Ru-Tuss II (Boots)
Triphenyl (Rugby)

Generic Available: yes

Type of Drug: respiratory decongestant and antihistamine

Used for: Treatment of allergies, hay fever, and nasal stuffiness, runny nose, and sneezing associated with the common cold.

How This Medication Works: Phenylpropanolamine causes the blood vessels to become smaller, which can relieve a stuffy nose or congestion. Chlorpheniramine prevents the effects of histamine—a substance produced in the body that causes sneezing, itching, and runny nose.

Dosage Form and Strength:
- tablets (25 mg phenylpropanolamine/4 mg chlorpheniramine, 37.5 mg/4 mg)
- sustained-release tablets (25 mg/4 mg)

- sustained-release capsules (75 mg/4 mg, 75 mg/8 mg, 75 mg/10 mg, 75 mg/12 mg)
- syrup (12.5 mg/2 mg per 5 mL)

Storage:
- room temperature
- protected from humidity

Administration:
- Take with food or milk if stomach upset occurs.
- To measure syrup, use a measuring device that can measure in milliliters (mL or ml); an ordinary teaspoon is not accurate enough.

Precautions:
Do not use if:
- you are allergic to phenylpropanolamine, chlorpheniramine, hydroxyzine, or other similar medications such as diphenhydramine, terfenadine, cyproheptadine, pseudoephedrine, phenylephrine, and epinephrine.

Talk to your doctor if:
- you have asthma, enlarged prostate, difficulty urinating, glaucoma, diabetes, kidney disease, liver disease, or thyroid disease.
- you are taking other medications such as those for heart disease or high blood pressure (hypertension), glaucoma, depression, infection (antibiotics), diabetes, thyroid disease, or weight loss.

Side Effects:
Major:
- skin rash, hives, or itching
- hallucinations or confusion

- drowsiness or feeling faint
- seizures or convulsions
- irregular heartbeat
- headache
- nausea or vomiting
- difficulty breathing
- sore throat or fever
- nervousness or restlessness

Minor:
- dizziness or light-headedness
- nightmares
- thickening of mucus
- blurred vision
- difficult or painful urination
- irregular heartbeat
- increased sensitivity to sun
- increased sweating
- increased appetite
- trouble sleeping

Time Required for Drug to Take Effect: Starts
to work within 15 to 30 minutes.

Symptoms of Overdose:
- nausea and vomiting
- seizures or convulsions
- irregular heartbeat
- nervousness or irritability
- dry mouth, throat, or nose
- flushed skin
- dilated pupils
- difficulty breathing
- severe dizziness or drowsiness

Special Notes:

- Check with your physician or pharmacist before using any over-the-counter medications.
- Tell your doctor you are taking this medication before you have skin tests for allergies.
- Do not drink alcohol or take medications that cause drowsiness or mental slowing.
- Avoid activities requiring mental alertness, such as operating a motor vehicle or machinery.
- If you experience dryness of the mouth, try sugarless candy or gum, ice chips, or a saliva substitute.
- Tell the doctor or dentist you are taking this medication before undergoing any treatment.
- Do not take diet-aids or medications for weight loss along with this medication.

phenytoin

Brand Name: Dilantin (Parke-Davis)

Generic Available: yes

Type of Drug: anticonvulsant

Used for: Prevention of seizures.

How This Medication Works: Alters the movement of the electrolyte sodium to interfere with abnormal electrical activity in the brain.

Dosage Form and Strength:

- tablet (50 mg)
- capsules (30 mg, 100 mg)
- oral suspension (30 mg/5 mL, 125 mg/5 mL)

Storage:
- room temperature
- tightly closed

Administration:
- Usually taken 3 times daily; certain brand name capsules may be taken once daily.
- Shake suspension well before each dose.
- Swallow capsule whole; do not crush or chew.
- Tablets may be crushed or chewed.
- If using antacids, separate doses of phenytoin and antacid by 2 hours.

Precautions:
Do not use if:
- you are allergic to phenytoin or other agents in the hydantoin family such as fosphenytoin.

Talk to your doctor if:
- you are taking any medication, especially allopurinol, benzodiazepines (such as diazepam or clonazepam), cimetidine, isoniazid, omeprazole, trimethoprim, valproic acid, salicylates (aspirin), tricyclic antidepressants (such as amitriptyline, imipramine, or desipramine), phenobarbital, carbamazepine, rifampin, theophylline, antacids, sucralfate, haloperidol, quinidine, theophylline, digoxin, amiodarone, doxycycline, and lithium.
- you have kidney disease, liver disease, or a fever.

Side Effects:
Major:
- bleeding or tender gums
- confusion, dizziness, or slurred speech
- rash

Minor:
- constipation
- drowsiness
- increased hair growth on face and body

Time Required for Drug to Take Effect:
Begins to work within hours and decreases the number and/or frequency of seizures as long as it is continued.

Symptoms of Overdose:
- blurred or double vision
- severe dizziness, drowsiness, or confusion

Special Notes:
- Regular dentist visits and good oral hygiene may help prevent or delay bleeding, tender gums.
- Do not discontinue without first talking with your doctor or pharmacist.
- Check with your physician or pharmacist before using any over-the-counter medications.
- You will occasionally have blood drawn to monitor the amount of phenytoin in your blood.

piroxicam

Brand Name: Feldene (Pratt)

Generic Available: no

Type of Drug: nonsteroidal anti-inflammatory drug (analgesic, anti-inflammatory, and antipyretic)

Used for: Relief of pain associated with osteoarthritis, rheumatoid and gouty arthritis, and surgical recovery.

How This Medication Works: Inhibits substances called prostaglandins that cause pain and inflammation.

Dosage Form and Strength: capsule (10 mg, 20 mg)

Storage:
- room temperature
- tightly closed
- protected from moisture and light

Administration:
- Usually taken once or twice daily.
- Take with meals or milk if stomach upset occurs.
- Do not lie down for at least 30 minutes after taking this medicine.
- Take with a full glass of water (6 to 8 ounces).

Precautions:
Do not use if:
- you are allergic to piroxicam or any other non-steroidal anti-inflammatory drugs such as ibuprofen, indomethacin, or aspirin.
- medicine is beyond the expiration date or unusual in appearance.

Talk to your doctor if:
- you are taking aspirin, another nonsteroidal anti-inflammatory drug (such as ibuprofen, indomethacin, or naproxen), anticoagulants (such as warfarin), steroids (such as prednisone), lithium, diuretics (such as furosemide or hydrochlorothiazide), methotrexate, or beta blockers (such as atenolol or propranolol).

- you have peptic ulcer disease, bleeding from your stomach or intestines, bleeding abnormalities, ulcerative colitis, high blood pressure (hypertension), kidney disease, liver disease, heart disease, asthma, or nasal polyps.
- you smoke tobacco or drink alcohol.

Side Effects:

Major:

- blood in stool or dark, tarry stool
- persistent or severe stomach or abdominal pain
- vomiting blood
- blood in urine or dark, smokey-colored urine
- difficulty urinating
- rash
- difficulty breathing
- swelling of the eyelids, throat, lips, or face
- vision or hearing changes
- unexplained sore throat or fever
- unusual bleeding or bruising
- irregular heartbeat

Minor:

- stomach upset, gas, or heartburn
- diarrhea or constipation
- swelling of hands or feet
- dizziness or drowsiness
- headache
- increased sensitivity to the sun or ultraviolet light

Time Required for Drug to Take Effect: Starts
to relieve pain in 1 to 2 hours. However, it may take 2 to 4 weeks to feel the full benefits of this medicine when treating arthritis.

Symptoms of Overdose:
- stomach pain, nausea, and vomiting
- heartburn
- gastrointestinal bleeding
- drowsiness or loss of consciousness
- headache
- confusion

Special Notes:
- Drinking alcohol or smoking increases your risk of bleeding from the stomach or intestines.
- Tell the doctor or dentist you are taking piroxicam if you are going to have surgery or emergency treatment.
- Contact your physician if pain or fever worsens during treatment.
- Use a sunblock with at least SPF 15 when outside because piroxicam may increase your sensitivity to the sun.

prazosin

Brand Name: Minipress (Pfizer)

Generic Available: yes

Type of Drug: antihypertensive

Used for: Treatment of high blood pressure (hypertension), enlarged prostate (benign prostatic hypertrophy), and Raynaud disease.

How This Medication Works: Dilates arteries and veins to lower blood pressure.

Dosage Form and Strength: capsules (1 mg, 2 mg, 5 mg)

Storage:
- room temperature
- tightly closed
- protected from humidity

Administration:
- Usually taken 2 to 3 times daily.
- Can be taken without regard to food.

Precautions:
Do not use if:
- you are allergic to prazosin, terazosin, or doxazosin.

Talk to your doctor if:
- you have congestive heart failure or severe kidney disease.
- you are taking a beta blocker (such as atenolol, metoprolol, or propranolol), clonidine, verapamil, or indomethacin.

Side Effects:
Major:
- fainting

Minor:
- dizziness or drowsiness
- headache
- fluid retention (edema)
- nausea
- palpitations

Time Required for Drug to Take Effect: Has its peak effect in 1 to 3 hours and lasts 10 to 12 hours.

Symptoms of Overdose:
- profound drowsiness and low blood pressure

Special Notes:
- Prazosin can cause extreme dizziness, especially when beginning therapy; take the first dose at bedtime, and avoid driving or hazardous tasks.
- Taking prazosin at bedtime (if prescribed once daily), will make the side effects of dizziness and sedation less bothersome.
- Changing positions slowly when sitting and/or standing up may help decrease dizziness.
- Prazosin is not a cure, and you may have to take this medication for a long time.

prednisone

Brand Names:
Deltasone (Upjohn)
Meticorten (Schering)
Orasone (Solvay)

Generic Available: yes

Type of Drug: hormone (adrenal cortical steroid)

Used for: Treatment of rheumatoid arthritis, lung diseases, lupus, ulcerative colitis, eye disorders, skin problems, poison ivy, and some cancers.

How This Medication Works: Prednisone is a cortisonelike substance naturally produced in the body. In most conditions the mechanism is unknown, but often the benefits are from decreasing inflammation.

Dosage Form and Strength:
- tablets (1 mg, 2.5 mg, 5 mg, 10 mg 20 mg, 25 mg, 50 mg)
- solution (5 mg/5 mL, 5 mg/mL)
- syrup (5 mg/5 mL)

Storage:
- room temperature
- tightly closed
- protected from light

Administration:
- If you are taking prednisone once daily, take it before 9:00 A.M.
- Take with food or milk if stomach upset occurs.
- If you miss a dose and you are taking it more than once daily, take the dose as soon as you remember it; if you do not remember until the next dose, double the dose and return to your regular schedule. If you are taking the dose once daily, take the dose as soon as you remember unless it is the next day; if it is the next day, do not double the dose; take your regular dose and return to your regular schedule. If you miss a dose taking it every other day, take the dose as soon as you remember it that day; if it is the day after the dose was to be taken, take it and start over on the every-other-day schedule, skipping the next day and taking it the following day. If you miss more than one dose, call your doctor.
- If you take the solution, it must be measured with a dropper or special medication-measuring spoon or cup; a kitchen spoon is not accurate enough.

Precautions:
Do not use if:
- you have had a serious allergic reaction to prednisone, dexamethasone, prednisolone, betamethasone, cortisone, dexamethasone, hydrocortisone, triamcinolone, or any other steroids.

Talk to your doctor if:
- you have bone disease, diabetes, emotional problems, glaucoma, fungal infections, heart disease, high blood pressure (hypertension), high cholesterol, kidney disease, liver disease, myasthenia gravis, stomach problems (ulcers or gastritis), thyroid disease, tuberculosis, or ulcerative colitis.
- you are taking any medication, especially aspirin or nonsteroidal anti-inflammatory drugs (such as ibuprofen or indomethacin), anticoagulants (such as warfarin), cholestyramine, colestipol, diabetes medications (such as insulin, glipizide, or tolbutamide), diuretics (such as hydrochlorothiazide or furosemide), seizure medications (such as phenobarbital or phenytoin), or tuberculosis medications (such as isoniazid or rifampin).

Side Effects:
Major:
- acne or other skin problems
- back or rib pain
- unusual or frequent bleeding or bruising
- bloody or black, tarry stools
- blurred vision, eye pain, or headaches
- fever or sore throat
- slow wound healing
- mood changes

- muscle weakness or wasting
- rapid weight gain (3 to 5 pounds in a week)
- seizures
- shortness of breath
- stomach enlargement or pain
- increased thirst
- increased urination

Minor:
- dizziness
- increased appetite
- indigestion
- increased sweating
- reddening of the skin on the face
- restlessness and sleep disorders

Time Required for Drug to Take Effect: Varies depending on the condition treated.

Symptoms of Overdose:
- agitation
- mania or psychotic behavior

Special Notes:
- Prednisone can cause low potassium levels. Talk to your doctor about making diet changes.
- You may need dosage adjustments during stressful times. Tell your doctor if you have a serious infection or injury or if you have to have surgery.
- If you are taking prednisone for long periods, it may cause glaucoma and cataracts.
- If you take prednisone for long periods, it may increase blood sugar and even cause diabetes.
- While you are taking prednisone, you should not receive live vaccinations or immunizations.

primidone

Brand Name: Mysoline (Wyeth-Ayerst)

Generic Available: yes

Type of Drug: anticonvulsant

Used for: Treatment of epilepsy.

How This Medication Works: Enhances the activity of the neurotransmitter gamma amino butyric acid to depress the central nervous system and prevent seizures. Primidone is also changed by the liver to phenobarbital and, therefore, also shares the activity of phenobarbital.

Dosage Form and Strength:
- tablets (50 mg, 250 mg)
- oral suspension (250 mg/5 mL)

Storage:
- room temperature
- tightly closed

Administration:
- Usually taken 3 to 4 times daily.
- Shake suspension well before taking.
- Take with food or milk if medication causes stomach upset.

Precautions:
Do not use if:
- you have had an allergic reaction to primidone, phenobarbital, or other medications of the barbiturate family.

Talk to your doctor if:
- you are taking any other medication, especially rifampin, valproic acid, warfarin, beta blockers (specifically propranolol and metoprolol), carbamazepine, clonazepam, corticosteroids (such as prednisone), doxycycline, felodipine, phenytoin, quinidine, theophylline, verapamil, or monamine oxidase (MAO) inhibitors (such as phenelzine and tranylcypromine).
- you have asthma, kidney disease, or liver disease.

Side Effects:
Major:
- excitement and restlessness

Minor:
- dizziness, drowsiness, or clumsiness
- nausea and vomiting

Time Required for Drug to Take Effect:
Therapy with this medication decreases the number and/or frequency of seizures as long as it is continued.

Symptoms of Overdose:
- confusion or double vision
- shortness of breath

Special Notes:
- This medication may cause drowsiness. Use caution when operating a motor vehicle or operating dangerous machinery.
- Do not drink alcohol while taking this medication.
- Check with your physician or pharmacist before using any over-the-counter medications.
- Do not discontinue without your doctor's consent.

procainamide

Brand Names:
Pronestyl (Princeton Pharm)
Procan SR (Parke-Davis)

Generic Available: yes

Type of Drug: antiarrhythmic

Used for: Treatment of abnormal heart rhythm (arrhythmia).

How This Medication Works: Stabilizes the cardiac muscle membrane, making the heart less excitable; prolongs the resting stage between electrical impulses; and decreases the speed of electrical conduction.

Dosage Form and Strength:
- capsules (250 mg, 375 mg, 500 mg)
- sustained-release tablets (250 mg, 500 mg, 750 mg, 1000 mg)

Storage:
- room temperature
- tightly closed
- protected from humidity

Administration:
- Usually taken 3 or 4 times daily.
- Take at even intervals.
- Do not crush or chew sustained-release tablets.
- Take with food or milk if stomach upset occurs.
- If you miss a dose, take as soon as possible. If it is close to the time for the next dose, do not take the missed dose. NEVER double your dose.

Precautions:

Do not use if:
- you are allergic to procainamide, procaine or other local anesthetic medications, tartrazine, or sulfites.
- medicine is beyond the expiration date.

Talk to your doctor if:
- you are taking other medications for abnormal heart rhythm (such as disopyramide or amiodarone), a beta blocker (such as atenolol, metoprolol, timolol, or propranolol), a histamine H_2 blocker for your stomach (such as cimetidine, nizatidine, ranitidine, or famotidine), or digoxin.
- you have congestive heart failure, liver disease, myasthenia gravis, lupus erythematosus, or kidney disease.

Side Effects:

Major:
- joint or muscle pain
- fever
- skin rash
- unexplained bruising or bleeding
- dark urine
- yellowing of the eyes (jaundice)
- chest pain
- hallucinations
- persistent diarrhea
- severe abdominal pain
- fainting

Minor:
- nausea and vomiting
- abdominal pain

- diarrhea
- dizziness

Time Required for Drug to Take Effect:
Begins to exert its effect in about half an hour and continue, to work for 3 or more hours. However, you must take this medication on a regular basis to prevent abnormal heart rhythms.

Symptoms of Overdose:
- life-threatening abnormal heart rhythms
- lethargy
- coma
- respiratory depression
- tremor

Special Notes:
- Your doctor will take blood tests to determine the amount of procainamide, and its major metabolite, NAPA, in your system.
- Taking procainamide as close as possible to the way it is prescribed is very important.
- Long-term use of procainamide can lead to a type of auto-immune disorder (lupus erythematosus–like syndrome). If you develop muscle or joint pain, fever, or a skin rash, contact your physician.
- Procainamide can cause a blood disorder called agranulocytosis, especially in the first 3 months of treatment. In agranulocytosis, the drug causes your body to stop producing infection-fighting white blood cells. Should you develop signs of infection (fever, sore throat, chills) call your doctor so that a complete blood count can be taken.

prochlorperazine

Brand Name: Compazine (SK Beecham)

Generic Available: yes

Type of Drug: antiemetic

Used for: Prevention or relief of severe nausea and vomiting.

How This Medication Works: Blocks the effects of the neurotransmitter dopamine, which is responsible for stimulating the vomiting center in the brain.

Dosage Form and Strength:
- tablets (5 mg, 10 mg, 25 mg)
- sustained-release capsules (10 mg, 15 mg, 30 mg)
- syrup (5 mg/5 mL)
- suppositories (2.5 mg, 5 mg, 25 mg)

Storage:
- room temperature
- tightly closed

Administration:
- Tablets usually taken 2 to 4 times daily.
- Capsules usually taken once or twice daily.
- Suppositories usually taken once or twice daily.
- Syrup usually taken 2 to 4 times daily.
- Do not open or crush the sustained-release capsules.
- To insert the suppository, you can moisten the tip with water; do not use anything else or it may reduce the effectiveness of the medicine.

Precautions:
Do not use if:
- you have ever had an allergic reaction to prochlorperazine.

Talk to your doctor if:
- you are taking medicines for Parkinson disease, seizures, depression, sleep problems, or anxiety.
- you have heart disease, liver disease, or glaucoma (angle closure type).

Side Effects:
Major:
- seizures
- stiff, rigid muscles
- fever
- difficulty breathing
- sweating
- loss of bladder control
- severe constipation
- eye pain
- change in vision
- severe agitation or restlessness
- severe rash

Minor:
- dizziness
- light-headedness
- drowsiness
- dry mouth
- mild constipation

Time Required for Drug to Take Effect: Relief
of symptoms can occur within 30 to 90 minutes, but may require a longer period of time.

Symptoms of Overdose:
- severe drowsiness or fainting
- severe agitation or restlessness
- palpitations

Special Notes:
- If vomiting is severe and not relieved by this medicine, you may become dehydrated, which is a serious problem; call your doctor for advice.
- If you use the syrup form of this medicine, take care to avoid contact with skin since it may cause irritation. If you get the medicine on your skin, wash the area well with water.
- Use a sunblock with at least SPF 15 when outside because prochlorperazine may increase your sensitivity to the sun.
- Do not drink alcohol while taking this medication.

promethazine

Brand Names:

Phenergan (Wyeth-Ayerst)

Phenergan Plain (Wyeth-Ayerst)

Phenameth (Major)

Prothazine (Vortech)

Phenergan Fortis (Wyeth-Ayerst)

Generic Available: yes

Type of Drug: antihistamine

Used for: Treatment of allergies, hay fever, hives, itching, sneezing or runny nose associated with the common cold, motion sickness, and watery, itchy eyes.

How This Medication Works: Prevents the
effects of histamine—a substance produced in the body
which causes sneezing, itching, and runny nose.

Dosage Form and Strength:
- tablets (12.5 mg, 25 mg, 50 mg)
- syrup (6.25 mg/5 mL, 25 mg/5 mL)
- suppositories (12.5 mg, 25 mg, 50 mg)

Storage:
Tablets and syrup:
- room temperature
- protected from humidity

Suppositories:
- refrigerated

Administration:
- Take each dose with a full glass of water.

Precautions:
Do not use if:
- you are allergic to promethazine or similar drugs
  such as diphenhydramine or chlorpheniramine.

Talk to your doctor if:
- you have emphysema, chronic bronchitis, asthma
  or other breathing problems; seizures or convulsions; gallbladder disease or gallstones; glaucoma; enlarged prostate; difficulty urinating; or
  kidney, liver or thyroid disease.
- you are taking any other medications.

Side Effects:
Major:
- skin rash, hives, or itching
- sore throat or fever

- hallucinations
- feeling faint
- seizures or convulsions
- difficulty breathing
- nervousness or restlessness

Minor:
- drowsiness or dizziness
- thickening of mucus
- blurred vision or confusion
- difficult or painful urination
- irregular heartbeat
- increased sensitivity to sun
- increased sweating
- increased appetite
- nightmares

Time Required for Drug to Take Effect: Starts to work within 20 minutes.

Symptoms of Overdose:
- dry mouth, throat, or nose
- flushed skin
- dilated pupils
- difficulty breathing
- severe dizziness or drowsiness
- excitation

Special Notes:
- Check with your physician or pharmacist before using any over-the-counter medications.
- Tell the doctor you are taking promethazine if you are going to have a skin test for allergies.
- Do not drink alcohol or take medications that cause drowsiness or mental slowing.

- Avoid activities requiring mental alertness, such as operating a motor vehicle or operating dangerous machinery.
- If you experience dryness of the mouth, try sugarless candy or gum, ice chips, or a saliva substitute.
- Tell the doctor or dentist you are taking promethazine if you are going to have surgery or emergency treatment.

promethazine and codeine combination

Brand Names:
Phenergan with Codeine (Wyeth-Ayerst)

Prothazine DC (Vortech)

Pherazine with Codeine (Halsey)

Generic Available: yes

Type of Drug: respiratory antihistamine and cough suppressant

Used for: Relief of symptoms of the common cold with runny nose and cough.

How This Medication Works: Promethazine prevents the effects of histamine—a substance produced in the body which causes sneezing, itching, runny nose. Codeine inhibits the cough center in the brain while decreasing the ability of the body to cough.

Dosage Form and Strength: liquid (6.25 mg promethazine/10 mg codeine per 5 mL)

Storage:
- room temperature
- protected from humidity

Administration:
- Take each dose with plenty of water.

Precautions:
Do not use if:
- you are allergic to promethazine or similar medications such as diphenhydramine, chlorpheniramine, or pheniramine.
- you are allergic to codeine or other narcotics such as morphine or hydrocodone.

Talk to your doctor if:
- you have emphysema, chronic bronchitis, asthma, or other breathing problems; seizures or convulsions; gallbladder disease or gallstones; glaucoma; enlarged prostate; difficulty urinating; or kidney, liver, or thyroid disease.
- you are taking any other medications.

Side Effects:
Major:
- skin rash, hives, or itching
- cold, clammy skin or flushed face
- confusion or hallucinations
- difficult or painful urination
- severe drowsiness or dizziness
- severe nervousness
- pinpoint pupils of eyes
- irregular heartbeat
- slowed or difficult breathing
- seizures or convulsions

Minor:
- constipation
- decreased sweating
- slight dizziness or light-headedness
- dryness of mouth, nose, or throat
- nausea or vomiting
- nightmares
- thickening of mucus
- unusual excitement, nervousness

Time Required for Drug to Take Effect: Starts to work within 20 minutes.

Symptoms of Overdose:
- difficulty breathing
- severe drowsiness, dizziness, or tiredness
- excitability or irritability
- dilated pupils

Special Notes:
- Check with your physician or pharmacist before using any over-the-counter medications.
- Tell the doctor you are taking this medication if you are going to have a skin test for allergies.
- Do not drink alcohol or take medications that cause drowsiness or mental slowing.
- Avoid activities requiring mental alertness, such as operating a motor vehicle or operating dangerous machinery.
- If you experience dryness of the mouth, try sugarless candy or gum, ice chips, or a saliva substitute.
- Tell the doctor or dentist you are taking this medication if you are going to have surgery or emergency treatment.

propoxyphene napsylate and acetaminophen combination

Brand Names:
Darvocet-N 50 (Lilly)   Propacet 100 (Lemmon)
Darvocet-N 100 (Lilly)

Generic Available: yes

Type of Drug: analgesic

Used for: Relief of pain.

How This Medication Works: Propoxyphene
acts in the central nervous system to decrease the recognition of pain impulses. Acetaminophen works in the peripheral nervous system and blocks pain impulses.

Dosage Form and Strength: tablets (50 mg
propoxyphene napsylate/325 mg acetaminophen, 100 mg/650 mg)

Storage:
- room temperature
- protected from humidity

Administration:
- Take with milk or food if medication causes stomach upset.
- Take this medication as prescribed and do not exceed the maximum number of doses per day. Each agent can be harmful if used in excess. Never take more tablets per dose than your doctor has prescribed.

Precautions:
Do not use if:
- you are allergic to propoxyphene or related medications such as methadone.
- you are allergic to acetaminophen.

Talk to your doctor if:
- you have alcoholism or other substance abuse problems; brain disease or head injury; colitis; seizures; emotional problems or mental illness; emphysema, asthma, or other lung diseases; kidney, liver, or thyroid disease; prostate problems or problems with urination; or gallbladder disease or gallstones.
- you are taking naltrexone, zidovudine, or any other medications, especially those that can cause drowsiness such as antihistamines, barbiturates (phenobarbital), benzodiazepines (diazepam, lorazepam), muscle relaxants, antidepressants, anticoagulants (warfarin), or carbamazepine.

Side Effects:
Major:
- skin rash or hives
- irregular breathing or difficulty breathing
- fast, slow, or pounding heartbeat
- painful or difficult urination
- frequent urge to urinate
- severe confusion or hallucinations
- depression
- pinpoint red spots on skin
- unusual bruising or bleeding
- trembling or uncontrolled muscle movements
- yellow eyes or skin (jaundice)

Minor:
- constipation
- drowsiness
- dry mouth
- general feeling of discomfort or illness
- loss of appetite
- nervousness, restlessness, or difficulty sleeping

Time Required for Drug to Take Effect: Starts
to work within 10 to 30 minutes and exerts its peak
effect after about 2 hours.

Symptoms of Overdose:
- cold, clammy skin
- seizures
- severe dizziness, drowsiness, or confusion
- continued nausea, vomiting, or diarrhea
- severe nervousness or restlessness
- difficulty breathing
- slowed heartbeat

(Symptoms associated with acetaminophen may not
occur until 2 to 4 days after the overdose is taken, but it
is important to begin treatment as soon as possible after
the overdose to prevent liver damage or death.)

Special Notes:
- This medication may cause drowsiness. Do not
  operate a motor vehicle or other machinery while
  you are taking this medication.
- Propoxyphene causes constipation. This side
  effect may be diminished by drinking 6 to 8 full
  glasses of water each day. If using this medication
  for chronic pain, adding a stool softener–laxative
  combination may be necessary.

- Check with your physician or pharmacist before using any over-the-counter medications.
- When propoxyphene is used over a long period of time, your body may become tolerant and require larger doses.
- Do not discontinue without your doctor's consent.
- Do not drink alcohol while taking this medication.
- Nausea and vomiting may occur, especially after the first few doses. This effect may go away if you lie down for a while.
- If you experience dryness of the mouth, try a sugarless candy or gum, ice chips, or a saliva substitute.
- If you think you or anyone else may have taken an overdose, get emergency help immediately.

propranolol

Brand Names:
Inderal (Wyeth-Ayerst)
Inderal LA (Wyeth-Ayerst)

Generic Available: yes

Type of Drug: antihypertensive (beta-adrenergic blocking agent [beta blocker])

Used for: Treatment of angina (chest pressure or discomfort), abnormal heart rhythms (arrhythmias), heart attacks, high blood pressure (hypertension), migraine headaches, and tremors of the hand.

How This Medication Works: Inhibits certain hormones that increase heart rate and blood pressure.

Dosage Form and Strength:
- tablets (10 mg, 20 mg, 40 mg, 60 mg, 80 mg, 90 mg)
- extended-release capsules (60 mg, 80 mg, 120 mg, 160 mg)

Storage:
- room temperature
- protected from humidity

Administration:
- Take at the same time every day.
- Swallow whole; do not crush or chew.

Precautions:
Do not use if:
- you have ever had an allergic reaction to propranolol or another beta blocker such as atenolol or metaprolol.

Talk to your doctor if:
- you are taking any other medications.

Side Effects:
Major:
- skin rash, itching
- sexual dysfunction
- difficulty breathing
- cold hands and feet
- confusion, hallucinations, nightmares
- palpitations or irregular heart beat
- depression
- swelling of feet, ankles, or lower legs
- chest pressure or discomfort
- unusual bleeding or bruising

Minor:
- nervousness, anxiety, or trouble sleeping
- low blood pressure (light-headedness, dizziness)
- drowsiness
- nausea, stomach upset, diarrhea, or constipation

Time Required for Drug to Take Effect: Starts to work within 1 to 2 hours. However, it takes at least 2 to 4 weeks to see the maximal response.

Symptoms of Overdose:
- slow, fast, or irregular heartbeat
- fainting or severe dizziness
- difficulty breathing
- seizures or convulsions
- blue tint to nail beds or palms

Special Notes:
- Do not discontinue without your doctor's consent.
- Propranolol is not a cure, and you may have to take this medication for a long time.
- Propranolol is used to prevent angina, and sublingual tablets (those placed under the tongue) may be required to treat or relieve an acute attack of angina.
- If you notice dizziness, avoid activities requiring mental alertness, such as operating a motor vehicle or dangerous machinery.
- Changing positions slowly when sitting and/or standing up may help decrease dizziness.
- Older patients may be more sensitive to cold temperatures while taking propranolol.
- Check with your physician or pharmacist before using any over-the-counter medications.

- Propranolol may slow the heart rate. Ask your doctor what your safe range is, but call your physician if your heart rate falls below 50 beats per minute.
- Be careful to avoid becoming dehydrated or overheated. Avoid saunas and strenuous exercise in hot weather, especially during the hot summer months, and avoid alcoholic beverages. Drink plenty of fluids to prevent dehydration during exercise and hot weather.

pseudoephedrine and guaifenesin combination

Brand Names:

Congess Sr (Fleming)
Respaire–60 SR (Laser)
Guaifed (Muro)
Respaire–120 SR (Laser)
Guaifed-PD (Muro)
Sinufed Timecelles (Roberts)
Versacaps (Seatrace)
Tuss-LA (Seatrace)
Robitussin-PE (Robins)
Halotussin PE (Halsey)
GuaiCough PE (Schein)
Guaituss PE Syrup (Barre-National)
Guaifed Syrup (Muro)
Fedahist Expectorant Syrup (Schwarz)
Congestac Caplets (Menley & James)
Guaitab (Muro)
Histalet X (Solvay)
V-Dec-M (Seatrace)
Deconsal II (Adams)
Entex PSE (Proctor & Gamble)
GuaiMax-D (Central)
Zephrex-LA (Bock)
Ru-Tuss DE (Boots)
Zephrex (Bock)

Generic Available: no

Type of Drug: decongestant and expectorant

Used for: Relief of stuffy nose, congestion, and cough associated with the common cold.

How This Medication Works: Pseudoephedrine causes the blood vessels to become smaller, which can relieve a stuffy nose or congestion. Guaifenesin loosens mucus or phlegm in the lungs.

Dosage Form and Strength:
- tablets (60 mg pseudoephedrine/400 mg guaifenesin, 120 mg/400 mg)
- extended-release tablets (120 mg/500 mg, 60 mg/600 mg, 120 mg/600 mg)
- extended-release capsules (60 mg/200 mg, 120 mg/250 mg, 60 mg/300 mg, 120 mg/500 mg)
- liquid (30 mg/100 mg per 5 mL, 30 mg/200 mg per 5 mL)

Storage:
- room temperature
- protected from humidity

Administration:
- Drink a glass of water with each dose.
- Swallow extended-release capsules and tablets whole; do not crush or chew.

Precautions:
Do not use if:
- you have an allergy to pseudoephedrine or guaifenesin or other similar medications such as

phenylpropanolamine, phenylephrine, or epinephrine.

Talk to your doctor if:
- you have heart disease, high blood pressure (hypertension), diabetes, glaucoma, kidney disease, liver disease, or thyroid disease.
- you are taking other medications, especially medication for heart disease, high blood pressure (hypertension), glaucoma, diabetes, thyroid disease, or weight loss.

Side Effects:

Major:
- skin rash, hives, or itching
- confusion or hallucinations
- drowsiness
- seizures or convulsions
- irregular heartbeat
- headache
- nausea or vomiting
- nervousness
- difficulty breathing

Minor:
- dizziness, light-headedness, or drowsiness
- nightmares or trouble sleeping

Time Required for Drug to Take Effect: Starts to work within 15 to 30 minutes.

Symptoms of Overdose:
- nausea and vomiting
- seizures or convulsions
- irregular heartbeat
- nervousness or irritability

Special Notes:
- Check with your physician or pharmacist before using any over-the-counter medications.
- Do not take diet-aids or medications for weight loss along with this medication.
- Drink plenty of water to help loosen mucus and phlegm in your lungs.
- If your cough has not improved within 7 days or if you have a high fever, skin rash, headache, or sore throat with a cough, contact your doctor.
- Tell your doctor or dentist that you are taking this medication before any surgery or emergency treatment.

quinidine

Brand Names:

Quinora (Key)
Quinidex Extentabs (Robins)
Quinalan (Lannett)

Quinaglute Duratabs (Berlex)
Cardioquin (Purdue-Frederick)

Generic Available: yes

Type of Drug: antiarrhythmic

Used for: Treatment of abnormal rhythm (arrhythmia), especially atrial fibrillation.

How This Medication Works: Stabilizes the cardiac muscle membrane, making the heart less excitable; prolongs the resting stage between electrical impulses; and decreases the speed of electrical conduction.

Dosage Form and Strength:
- tablets (200 mg, 275 mg, 300 mg)
- extended-release tablets (300 mg, 324 mg)

Storage:
- room temperature
- tightly closed
- protected from humidity

Administration:
- Usually taken 3 or 4 times daily; sustained-release products may be taken twice daily.
- Take with food to minimize stomach upset.
- Swallow sustained-release tablets whole; do not crush or chew.
- If using antacids, separate doses of quinidine and antacid by 2 hours.

Precautions:
Do not use if:
- you are allergic to quinidine.
- medicine is beyond the expiration date.

Talk to your doctor if:
- you are taking other medications for abnormal heart rhythm (such as disopyramide, procainamide, or amiodarone), a tricyclic antidepressant (such as amitriptyline, desipramine, nortriptyline, or imipramine), cimetidine, phenytoin, nifedipine, rifampin, sucralfate, phenobarbital, verapamil, a beta blocker (such as atenolol, metoprolol, timolol, or propranolol), digoxin, or an anticoagulant (such as warfarin).
- you have ever had liver disease.
- you have congestive heart failure.

Side Effects:

Major:
- ringing in the ears (tinnitus)
- visual disturbances
- extreme dizziness or fainting
- severe headache
- skin rash
- difficulty breathing
- persistent diarrhea
- unexplained bruising or bleeding

Minor:
- headache
- dizziness
- diarrhea
- nausea, vomiting, and abdominal pain

Time Required for Drug to Take Effect:

Begins to exert its effect in about half an hour, and continues to work for 6 to 8 hours.

Symptoms of Overdose:

- confusion
- lethargy
- coma
- respiratory arrest
- seizures

Special Notes:

- Your doctor will take blood tests to determine the amount of quinidine in your system and your blood count, liver function, and kidney function.
- Use a sunblock with at least SPF 15 when outside because quinidine may increase your sensitivity to the sun.

ranitidine

Brand Name: Zantac (Glaxo Wellcome)

Generic Available: no

Type of Drug: gastrointestinal (histamine H_2 antagonist)

Used for: Treatment of excess acid production in the stomach, ulcers, and heartburn (gastroesophageal reflux disease [GERD]).

How This Medication Works: Blocks the binding of histamine to sites in the stomach that would cause acid secretion.

Dosage Form and Strength:
- tablets (150 mg, 300 mg)
- syrup (15 mg/mL)

Storage:
- room temperature
- protected from humidity

Administration:
- If you are taking multiple doses daily, take with or immediately after meals unless your doctor has different instructions.
- If you are only taking 1 dose daily, it is best to take it before bedtime unless your doctor has different instructions.
- Do not take antacids at the same time as ranitidine. Take ranitidine at least 2 hours after taking antacids or 1 hour before taking antacids.

Precautions:

Do not use if:
- you are allergic to ranitidine, cimetidine, famotidine, or nizatidine.

Talk to your doctor if:
- you have kidney or liver disease.
- you are taking any other medications, especially theophylline, anticoagulants (such as warfarin), antidepressants (such as amitriptyline, fluoxetine, or trazodone), antibiotics, phenytoin, or medications for heart disease or high blood pressure.

Side Effects:

Major:
- skin rash, hives, or itching
- blurred vision and confusion
- irregular heartbeat and tightness in the chest
- fever or sore throat
- swelling of eyelids
- unusual bleeding or bruising

Minor:
- constipation or diarrhea
- decreased sexual ability or desire
- dizziness or drowsiness
- headache
- dry mouth
- increased sweating
- joint or muscle pain
- loss of appetite
- nausea or vomiting
- ringing or buzzing in the ears (tinnitus)
- swelling of breasts (in men and women)
- hair loss

Time Required for Drug to Take Effect: Starts
to work within 1 to 3 hours, but ulcer healing may
require 4 to 12 weeks of therapy.

Symptoms of Overdose:
- difficulty breathing
- irregular heartbeat
- tremors
- vomiting or diarrhea
- light-headedness

Special Notes:
- Check with your physician or pharmacist before
  using any over-the-counter medications.
- Avoid medications that may make your ulcer
  worse, including nonsteroidal anti-inflammatory
  drugs (such as aspirin, ibuprofen, and naproxen).
- If you smoke, you should quit. If you continue to
  smoke, you should try not to smoke after the last
  dose of ranitidine for the day.
- This medication may cause drowsiness. Use
  caution when operating a motor vehicle or dangerous machinery.
- Avoid alcohol or other medications that may
  make you drowsy or dizzy, such as antihistamines, sedatives, tranquilizers, pain relievers,
  seizure medications, and muscle relaxants.
- Tell the doctor you are taking ranitidine if you are
  going to have a skin test for allergies.
- If you experience dryness of the mouth, try sugarless candy or gum, ice chips, or a saliva substitute.
- Tell the doctor or dentist you are taking ranitidine
  before undergoing any treatment.

rifampin

Brand Names:
Rimactane (Ciba-Geigy)
Rifadin (Marion Merrell Dow)

Generic Available: no

Type of Drug: anti-infective

Used for: Prevention of infection in persons exposed to tuberculosis; treatment of active tuberculosis, meningitis, and other serious infections, including Legionnaire disease, endocarditis, osteomyelitis, and prostatitis.

How This Medication Works: Kills bacteria by interfering with a bacterial protein produced by DNA (RNA polymerase).

Dosage Form and Strength: capsules (150 mg, 300 mg)

Storage:
- room temperature
- tightly closed
- protected from humidity
- protected from light

Administration:
- Usually taken once daily; dosage will depend on infection being treated.
- Take at about the same time everyday.
- Best if taken on an empty stomach.
- Take until completely gone, even if symptoms have improved.

- For tuberculosis treatment, continuous administration for several months is an important part of treatment; relapse rates are much higher if rifampin is stopped prematurely.

Precautions:

Do not use if:
- you are allergic to rifampin or rifamycin.
- medicine is beyond the expiration date.

Talk to your doctor if:
- you have ever had liver disease.
- you are taking medicines for the heart (such as verapamil, digoxin, or quinidine), an anticoagulant (such as warfarin), estrogen, steroids (such as prednisone or methylprednisolone), phenobarbital, diazepam, theophylline, a beta blocker (such as propranolol, atenolol, or metoprolol), an antifungal agent (such as ketoconazole), probenecid, or oral diabetes medication (such as glyburide or glipizide).
- you get another infection or this infection does not get better.

Side Effects:

Major:
- persistent diarrhea
- confusion
- behavioral changes
- unexplained bruising or bleeding

Minor:
- stomach upset, nausea, or vomiting
- heartburn
- loss of appetite

- abdominal cramps, flatulence, and diarrhea
- red-orange tears, sweat, saliva, urine, or feces
- headache

Time Required for Drug to Take Effect:
Begins to kill infecting bacteria within hours after taking your first dose. However, you must continue to take rifampin for the full course of treatment, even if symptoms disappear.

Symptoms of Overdose:
- nausea and vomiting
- lethargy
- loss of consciousness
- yellowing of skin or eyes (jaundice)

Special Notes:
- Do not use for infections other than the one for which it was prescribed.
- Rifampin may cause tears, sweat, saliva, urine, feces, and phlegm to turn red-orange in color. This may cause permanent discoloration of soft contact lenses.
- Your doctor will take blood tests to monitor your liver function if you are on rifampin for a prolonged course of treatment.

rimantadine

Brand Name: Flumadine (Forest)

Generic Available: no

Type of Drug: anti-infective

Used for: Prevention of infections after exposure to influenza A and treatment of influenza A.

How This Medication Works: Mechanism is not entirely understood, but appears to stop viral replication early in its cycle.

Dosage Form and Strength:
- tablets (100 mg)
- syrup (50 mg/5 mL)

Storage:
- room temperature
- tightly closed
- protected from humidity

Administration:
- The usual dose is 100 mg twice daily.
- Take until completely gone, even if symptoms have improved.

Precautions:
Do not use if:
- you are allergic to rimantadine or amantadine.
- medicine is beyond the expiration date.

Talk to your doctor if:
- you have ever had liver disease.
- you have kidney disease or a seizure disorder.
- you take acetaminophen, aspirin, or cimetidine.

Side Effects:
Major:
- seizures or hallucinations
- persistent diarrhea or vomiting
- agitation or inability to concentrate

Minor:
- nausea and vomiting
- abdominal pain, flatulence, or diarrhea
- nervousness
- insomnia

Time Required for Drug to Take Effect: If
taken within 48 hours of the first signs of influenza A, it decreases the severity and duration of symptoms. If taken before exposure to influenza A, it can prevent symptoms.

Symptoms of Overdose:
- agitation
- hallucinations
- cardiac arrhythmia

Special Notes:
- Do not use for infections other than the one for which it was prescribed.

risperidone

Brand Name: Risperdal (Janssen)

Generic Available: no

Type of Drug: antipsychotic

Used for: Treatment of psychotic disorders such as schizophrenia.

How This Medication Works: Mechanism is unknown but it may block the activity of the neurotransmitters dopamine and serotonin.

Dosage Form and Strength: tablets (1 mg, 2 mg, 3 mg, 4 mg)

Storage:
- room temperature
- protected from light

Administration:
- Usually taken 2 times daily.

Precautions:
Do not use if:
- you have ever had an allergic reaction to risperidone.
- you have Parkinson disease.

Talk to your doctor if:
- you are taking any other medications.
- you have heart problems, seizures, kidney disease, or liver disease.

Side Effects:
Major:
- restlessness or insomnia
- blurred vision or dizziness
- muscle spasms
- twitching movements
- rash or sunburn

Minor:
- fatigue
- constipation or diarrhea
- cough
- dry mouth
- headache
- drowsiness

Time Required for Drug to Take Effect: This medication may need to be taken for several weeks before desired effect is seen.

Symptoms of Overdose:
- drowsiness
- seizures
- increased heart rate

Special Notes:
- Do not drink alcohol while taking this medication.
- Changing positions slowly when sitting and/or standing up may help decrease dizziness caused by this medication.
- Do not discontinue without first talking with your doctor.
- Use a sunblock with at least SPF 15 when outside because risperidone may increase your sensitivity to the sun.

salicylate salts

Brand Names:
Arthropan (choline salicylate) (Purdue-Frederick)
Trilisate (choline magnesium trisalicylate) (Purdue-Frederick)

Generic Available: yes

Type of Drug: nonsteroidal anti-inflammatory drug (analgesic, anti-inflammatory, and antipyretic)

Used for: Treatment of musculoskeletal aches and pains and fever.

How This Medication Works: Inhibits substances called prostaglandins that cause pain and inflammation. Treats a fever by increasing heat loss from the body.

Dosage Form and Strength:
Choline salicylate:
- liquid/oral solution (870 mg/mL)

Choline magnesium trisalicylate:
- tablets (293 mg choline salicylate/362 mg magnesium salicylate, 440 mg/544 mg)
- liquid/oral solution (293 mg/362 mg per 5 mL)

Storage:
- room temperature
- tightly closed
- protected from humidity and sunlight

Administration:
- Usually taken 4 to 6 times daily.
- Take with meals or milk to minimize stomach upset.
- Do not lie down for at least 30 minutes after taking this medicine.
- Take with a full glass of water (6 to 8 ounces).

Precautions:
Do not use if:
- you are allergic to choline and magnesium salicylate or any other nonsteroidal anti-inflammatory drug such as ibuprofen, indomethacin, piroxicam, or aspirin.
- medicine is beyond the expiration date or unusual in appearance.

Talk to your doctor if:
- you are taking aspirin; another nonsteroidal anti-inflammatory drug such as ibuprofen, indomethacin, or piroxicam; anticoagulants such as warfarin; steroids such as prednisone; oral diabetes medication such as glipizide or glyburide; or methotrexate.
- you have peptic ulcer disease, bleeding from your stomach or intestines, bleeding abnormalities, ulcerative colitis, kidney disease, or liver disease.
- you smoke tobacco or drink alcohol.

Side Effects:
Major:
- blood in stool or dark, tarry stool
- persistent or severe stomach or abdominal pain
- vomiting blood
- blood in urine or dark, smokey-colored urine
- difficulty urinating
- rash
- difficulty breathing
- swelling of the eyelids, throat, lips, or face
- vision or hearing changes
- unusual bleeding or bruising

Minor:
- stomach upset, gas, or heartburn
- dizziness or drowsiness
- headache

Time Required for Drug to Take Effect: Starts
to relieve pain in 1 to 2 hours. However, it may take 2 to 4 weeks to feel the full benefits of this medicine when treating arthritis.

Symptoms of Overdose:
- stomach pain
- heartburn
- nausea and vomiting
- drowsiness
- headache
- confusion
- loss of consciousness
- gastrointestinal bleeding
- dehydration
- seizures

Special Notes:
- Drinking alcohol or smoking tobacco may increase your risk of bleeding from the stomach or intestines while taking choline and magnesium salicylate.
- Use a sunblock with at least SPF 15 when outside because choline and magnesium salicylate may increase your sensitivity to the sun.
- Tell the doctor or dentist you are taking choline and magnesium salicylate if you are going to have surgery or emergency treatment.
- Check with your physician before self-medicating with choline salicylate.
- Self-medication of fever with nonprescription choline salicylate should not exceed 3 days unless otherwise directed by a physician or pharmacist.
- Self-medication of pain with nonprescription choline salicylate should not exceed 10 days unless otherwise directed by a physician or pharmacist.

- If you have diabetes, large doses of salicylate salts may alter your blood sugar levels. Check with your doctor before you make any changes in your diabetes regimen.
- Contact physician if pain worsens during treatment.

salmeterol

Brand Name: Serevent (Schering)

Generic Available: no

Type of Drug: bronchodilator

Used for: Treatment of asthma.

How This Medication Works: Causes the passageways in the lungs to dilate.

Dosage Form and Strength: inhaler (21 µg/inhalation)

Storage:
- room temperature
- protected from humidity

Administration:
- Shake the canister well before using.
- Have your doctor or pharmacist demonstrate the proper procedure for using your inhaler and practice your technique in front of them.
- Allow at least 2 minutes between inhalations (puffs).
- If you have more than one inhaler, it is important to administer your inhalers in the correct order. If

you are using salmeterol and another inhaler, use the salmeterol first. Wait at least 5 minutes before inhaling the second medication.

Precautions:
Do not use if:
- you have had an allergic reaction to salmeterol, albuterol, epinephrine, metaproterenol, or terbutaline.

Talk to your doctor if:
- you have diabetes, heart disease, high blood pressure (hypertension), problems with circulation or blood vessels, seizures, convulsions, or thyroid disease.
- you are taking any other medications, especially medications for heart disease, high blood pressure (hypertension), migraines, or depression.

Side Effects:
Major:
- skin rash, itching, or hives
- wheezing or difficulty breathing
- bluish coloring of your skin
- swelling of face, lips, or eyelids
- fainting or dizziness
- chest discomfort or pressure
- irregular heartbeat
- numbness or tingling in hands or feet
- hallucinations

Minor:
- nervousness, tremor, trembling, or insomnia
- coughing
- dryness or irritation of mouth or throat

- unpleasant taste
- flushing or redness of face
- headache
- increased sweating
- muscle cramps or twitching
- nausea or vomiting
- drowsiness

Time Required for Drug to Take Effect: Starts to work within 20 minutes, and continues to work for 12 hours.

Symptoms of Overdose:
- chest discomfort or pressure
- chills or fever
- seizures or convulsions
- irregular heartbeat
- severe nausea or vomiting
- severe trouble breathing
- severe tremor or trembling
- blurred vision
- unusual paleness and coldness of skin

Special Notes:
- Salmeterol should not be used for acute asthma attacks.
- Check with your physician or pharmacist before using any over-the-counter medications.
- Sometimes a spacer device is used with your inhaler. A spacer device helps the medication get to the lungs instead of the mouth or throat.
- Keep track of how many inhalations are left and get your medication refilled about 1 week before you expect to run out.

salsalate

Brand Name: Disalcid (3M)

Generic Available: yes

Type of Drug: nonsteroidal anti-inflammatory drug (analgesic, anti-inflammatory, and antipyretic)

Used for: Treatment of musculoskeletal aches and pains and fever.

How This Medication Works: Inhibits substances called prostaglandins that cause pain and inflammation. Treats fever by increasing heat loss from the body.

Dosage Form and Strength:
- tablets (500 mg, 750 mg)
- capsules (500 mg)

Storage:
- room temperature
- tightly closed
- protected from humidity and sunlight

Administration:
- Usually taken 2 to 3 times daily, depending on the condition being treated.
- Take with meals or milk to minimize stomach upset.
- Do not lie down for at least 30 minutes after taking this medicine.
- Take medication with a full glass of water (6 to 8 ounces).

Precautions:
Do not use if:
- you are allergic to salsalate or any other non-steroidal anti-inflammatory drug such as ibuprofen, indomethacin, piroxicam, or aspirin.
- medicine is beyond the expiration date or is unusual in appearance.

Talk to your doctor if:
- you are taking aspirin; another nonsteroidal anti-inflammatory drug such as ibuprofen, indomethacin, or piroxicam; anticoagulants such as warfarin; steroids such as prednisone; oral diabetes medication such as glipizide or glyburide; or methotrexate.
- you have peptic ulcer disease, bleeding from your stomach or intestines, bleeding abnormalities, ulcerative colitis, kidney disease, or liver disease.
- you smoke tobacco or drink alcohol.

Side Effects:
Major:
- blood in stool or dark, tarry stool
- persistent or severe stomach or abdominal pain
- vomiting blood
- blood in urine or dark, smokey-colored urine
- difficulty urinating
- difficulty breathing
- rash or swelling of the eyelids, throat, lips, or face
- vision or hearing changes
- unusual bleeding or bruising

Minor:
- stomach upset, gas, or heartburn
- swelling of the hands or feet

Time Required for Drug to Take Effect: Starts
to relieve pain in 1 to 4 hours. However, it may take
2 to 4 weeks to feel the full benefits of this medicine
when treating arthritis.

Symptoms of Overdose:
- stomach pain
- heartburn
- nausea and vomiting
- drowsiness
- headache
- confusion
- loss of consciousness
- kidney failure
- gastrointestinal bleeding
- dehydration
- seizures

Special Notes:
- Drinking alcohol or smoking tobacco may
  increase your risk of bleeding from the stomach
  or intestines while taking salsalate.
- Use a sunblock with at least SPF 15 when outside
  because salsalate may increase your sensitivity to
  the sun.
- Tell the doctor or dentist you are taking salsalate
  if you are going to have surgery or emergency
  treatment.
- If you have diabetes, large doses of salsalate may
  alter your blood sugar levels. Check with your
  doctor before you make any changes in your diabetes regimen.
- Contact physician if pain worsens during treatment.

selegiline

Brand Name: Eldepryl (Somerset)

Generic Available: no

Type of Drug: antiparkinsonian (monoamine oxidase B [MAO-B] inhibitor)

Used for: Treatment of Parkinson disease.

How This Medication Works: Prolongs the action of the neurotransmitter dopamine in the brain by interfering with the enzyme—monoamine oxidase B (MAO-B)—that is responsible for metabolizing, or breaking down, dopamine.

Dosage Form and Strength: tablets (5 mg)

Storage:
- room temperature
- tightly closed

Administration:
- Usually taken once or twice daily.
- Take in the morning and at noon (if prescribed twice daily).

Precautions:
Do not use if:
- you have ever had an allergic reaction to selegiline.
- you are taking meperidine.

Talk to your doctor if:
- you are taking antidepressants, metoclopramide, or antipsychotics such as haloperidol or thioridazine.
- you have ever been treated for peptic ulcers.

Side Effects:

Major:
- chest pain
- palpitations
- unusually severe headache
- light sensitivity
- severe nausea or vomiting
- inability to urinate
- severe, painful constipation
- black, tarry stools
- unusual changes in behavior or thinking

Minor:
- light-headedness
- dizziness
- insomnia
- unusual movements
- unusual sweating
- constipation
- urinary problems

Time Required for Drug to Take Effect: Mild
improvement in symptoms may be noted within several days, but it may take weeks to see the optimum improvement.

Symptoms of Overdose:
- unusually low or high blood pressure
- fainting
- dizziness and falling
- unusual changes in behavior or memory
- unusual agitation or irritability
- severe muscle spasms
- seizures

Special Notes:
- Selegiline may be prescribed to slow Parkinson disease, although this benefit is still controversial.
- Do not exceed the recommended dose of selegiline.
- When selegiline is added to a regimen that includes levodopa, it may be necessary to reduce the dose of levodopa.
- Do not drink alcohol while taking this medication.
- Selegiline was formerly called L-deprenyl.

sertraline

Brand Name: Zoloft (Pfizer)

Generic Available: no

Type of Drug: antidepressant (selective serotonin reuptake inhibitor)

Used for: Treatment of depression and obsessive compulsive disorder.

How This Medication Works: Prolongs the effects of the neurotransmitter serotonin by interfering with its reuptake into nerve cells in the brain; also prolongs the actions of other neurotransmitters, such as epinephrine and dopamine but, to a much lesser extent.

Dosage Form and Strength: tablets (50 mg, 100 mg)

Storage:
- room temperature
- tightly closed

Administration:
- Usually taken once daily in the morning or at bedtime (if you experience drowsiness.)

Precautions:
Do not use if:
- you have ever had an allergic reaction to sertraline or other selective serotonin reuptake inhibitors such as fluvoxamine or paroxetine.
- you are currently taking, or have taken in the last 14 days, a monoamine oxidase (MAO) inhibitor such as phenelzine or tranylcypromine.

Talk to your doctor if:
- you have ever had liver problems, kidney problems, or seizures.
- you are taking benzodiazepines (such as alprazolam or diazepam), lithium, desipramine, warfarin, or tolbutamide.

Side Effects:
Major:
- rash, hives, or itching
- fever
- unusual agitation, restlessness, or excitement
- dizziness or fainting when standing up
- chest pain

Minor:
- headache
- agitation or sleeping problems
- drowsiness or dizziness
- vivid dreams
- tremor
- fatigue or weakness

- decreased sexual interest and function
- stomach pain, nausea, or diarrhea
- dry mouth
- sweating
- blurred vision
- urinary problems

Time Required for Drug to Take Effect: May
start to improve some symptoms within the first few weeks, but the full benefit may take from 4 to 8 weeks.

Symptoms of Overdose:
- severe agitation or excited behavior
- palpitations or chest pain

Special Notes:
- Know which "target symptoms" (restlessness, worry, fear, or changes in sleep or appetite) you are being treated for and be prepared to tell your doctor if your target symptoms are improving, worsening, or unchanged.
- Do not drink alcohol while taking this medication.
- Never increase your dose without the advice of your doctor.
- Do not discontinue without first talking with your doctor.

simvastatin

Brand Name: Zocor (Merck)

Generic Available: no

Type of Drug: antihyperlipidemic

Used for: Treatment of high blood cholesterol levels and cardiovascular atherosclerosis.

How This Medication Works: Decreases the amount of cholesterol manufactured in the liver by inhibiting an enzyme.

Dosage Form and Strength: tablets (5 mg, 10 mg, 20 mg, 40 mg)

Storage:
- room temperature
- tightly closed
- protected from humidity

Administration:
- Usually taken once daily.
- May be taken without regard to food.

Precautions:

Do not use if:
- you are allergic to simvastatin or similar drugs such as fluvastatin, lovastatin, or pravastatin.

Talk to your doctor if:
- you have liver disease.
- you are taking any other medication, especially cyclosporine, erythromycin, warfarin, niacin, or gemfibrozil.

Side Effects:

Major:
- unexplained muscle aches, especially if accompanied by malaise
- breathing difficulty
- swelling of the face, throat, lips, or tongue

Minor:
- insomnia
- abdominal pain or cramps
- diarrhea
- headache
- dizziness
- taste disturbances

Time Required for Drug to Take Effect: Starts lowering blood cholesterol levels in 1 to 2 weeks, but it may take 4 to 6 weeks to reach maximum effectiveness.

Symptoms of Overdose: no specific symptoms

Special Notes:
- After beginning therapy, your doctor will recheck your cholesterol levels in 1 to 3 months.
- Use a sunblock with at least SPF 15 when outside because simvastatin may increase your sensitivity to the sun.
- Do not drink alcohol while taking this medication.
- Reduce your dietary cholesterol intake.
- Simvastatin is not a cure and must be taken on a long-term basis to have an effect.
- Your doctor will monitor your liver function with laboratory blood work during therapy.

spironolactone

Brand Name: Aldactone (Searle)

Generic Available: yes

Type of Drug: diuretic

Used for: Treatment of fluid retention (edema), high blood pressure (hypertension), and hyperaldosteronism, and treatment and prevention of low potassium levels (hypokalemia) in patients taking digoxin.

How This Medication Works: Inhibits the formation of a protein necessary for sodium transport in the kidney, resulting in loss of water through urine.

Dosage Form and Strength: tablets (25 mg, 50 mg, 100 mg)

Storage:
- room temperature
- tightly closed
- protected from humidity

Administration:
- Usually taken 2 to 3 times daily.
- Take with food to increase absorption.

Precautions:
Do not use if:
- you are allergic to spironolactone.

Talk to your doctor if:
- you have kidney disease.
- you are taking triamterene, amiloride, warfarin, digoxin, potassium supplements, an angiotensin-converting enzyme inhibitor (such as captopril or enalapril), or a salicylate (such as aspirin).

Side Effects:
Major:
- seizures
- chest pain

- irregular heartbeat (very fast or very slow)
- skin rash

Minor:
- dry mouth
- drowsiness
- headache
- impotence
- enlargement of the breasts (in men and women)
- hair growth

Time Required for Drug to Take Effect: Starts
acting very gradually, with maximum effect after 3 days
of therapy.

Symptoms of Overdose:
- nausea and vomiting
- diarrhea
- profound muscle weakness

Special Notes:
- Avoid salt substitutes containing potassium.
  Spironolactone may cause your body to retain
  potassium.
- Your doctor will check your blood count, kidney
  function, and electrolyte (sodium, potassium)
  levels periodically during therapy.
- Unless otherwise instructed by your doctor, it is
  important to drink 6 to 8 eight-ounce glasses of
  water everyday. This will help avoid dehydration.
- Use a sunblock with at least SPF 15 when outside
  because spironolactone may increase your sensitivity to the sun.
- If you experience dryness of the mouth, try sugarless candy or gum, ice chips, or a saliva substitute.

- Weigh yourself daily. If you gain or lose more than 1 pound per day, call your doctor.
- Changing positions slowly when sitting and/or standing up may help decrease dizziness.
- If you notice dizziness, avoid activities requiring mental alertness, such as operating a motor vehicle or dangerous machinery.
- Do not drink alcohol while taking this medication.

sucralfate

Brand Name: Carafate (Marion Merrell Dow)

Generic Available: no

Type of Drug: gastrointestinal

Used for: Treatment of ulcers.

How This Medication Works: Forms a barrier, or coating, over the ulcer site, preventing stomach acid from further damaging the ulcer site.

Dosage Form and Strength: tablets (1 g)

Storage:
- room temperature
- protected from humidity

Administration:
- Take sucralfate 1 hour before meals or on an empty stomach.
- Take with plenty of water.
- If using antacids, separate doses of sucralfate and antacid by 1 hour.

Precautions:

Do not use if:
- you are allergic to sucralfate.

Talk to your doctor if:
- you have kidney disease or problems with your esophagus, swallowing, stomach, or intestines.
- you are taking any other drugs, especially antibiotics, digoxin, theophylline, phenytoin, antacids, cimetidine, ranitidine, nizatidine, or famotidine.

Side Effects:

Major:
- skin rash, hives, or itching
- seizures or convulsions
- drowsiness

Minor:
- dizziness
- nausea, stomach upset, diarrhea, or constipation
- backache
- dry mouth

Time Required for Drug to Take Effect: Binds
toulcer site within 1 to 2 hours. However, healing may require 4 to 12 weeks of therapy.

Symptoms of Overdose:
- seizures or convulsions
- drowsiness

Special Notes:
- Take for as long as directed even if symptoms have improved.
- Check with your physician or pharmacist before using any over-the-counter medications.

sulfamethoxazole and trimethoprim combination

Brand Names:

Bactrim (Roche)

Bactrim DS (Roche)

Septra (Burroughs
  Wellcome)

Septra DS (Burroughs
  Wellcome)

Cotrim (Lemmon)

Generic Available: yes

Type of Drug: anti-infective (sulfonamide)

Used for: Treatment of infections of the ear, respiratory tract, skin, and genitourinary tract.

How This Medication Works: Kills bacteria by inhibiting the bacteria's production of vital nucleic acids and proteins.

Dosage Form and Strength:

- tablets (80 mg trimethoprim/400 mg sulfamethoxazole, 160 mg/800 mg)
- suspension (40 mg/200 mg per 5 mL)

Storage:

- room temperature
- tightly closed
- protected from humidity

Administration:

- Usually taken twice daily, but dose and length of treatment will vary depending on the infection being treated.

- Take at even intervals (such as every 12 hours) and at the same time every day.
- Shake suspension well before measuring dose.
- Take each dose with a full glass of water.
- Best if taken on an empty stomach, but if stomach upset occurs, take with food or milk.
- Take until completely gone, even if symptoms have improved.

Precautions:

Do not use if:
- you are allergic to sulfamethoxazole, trimethoprim, or sulfa.
- medicine is beyond the expiration date.

Talk to your doctor if:
- you are taking an anticoagulant (such as warfarin), a diuretic (such as furosemide or hydrochlorothiazide), cyclosporine, dapsone, methotrexate, phenytoin, zidovudine, or an oral diabetes medication (such as glyburide or glipizide).
- you have kidney disease.

Side Effects:

Major:
- yellowing of the skin or eyes (jaundice)
- rash or hives
- unexplained bruising or bleeding
- sore throat, fever, or chills
- persistent vomiting or convulsions
- inability to walk or other impaired motor function

Minor:
- stomach upset, nausea, or vomiting
- headache

- abdominal pain
- mouth sores

Time Required for Drug to Take Effect:
Begins to kill infecting bacteria within hours. However, you must continue to take this medication for the full course of treatment, even if symptoms disappear.

Symptoms of Overdose:
- nausea or vomiting
- dizziness
- unconsciousness

Special Notes:
- Do not use for infections other than the one for which it was prescribed.
- Long-term treatment may lead to bacteria and fungus not sensitive to a sulfamethoxazole and trimethoprim combination.
- Use a sunblock with at least SPF 15 when outside because this medication may increase your sensitivity to the sun.
- Call your doctor if you get another infection or this infection does not get better.

sulfasalazine

Brand Names:
Azulfidine (Pharmacia)
Azulfidine EN-Tabs (Pharmacia)

Generic Available: yes

Type of Drug: anti-infective (sulfonamide)

Used for: Treatment of Crohn disease, ulcerative colitis, and rheumatoid arthritis.

How This Medication Works: The exact mechanism of sulfasalazine is not known, but components may have an anti-inflammatory and antibacterial effect on the lining of the large intestine.

Dosage Form and Strength:
- tablets (500 mg)
- enteric-coated tablets (500 mg)
- suspension (250 mg/5 mL)

Storage:
- room temperature
- tightly closed
- protected from humidity

Administration:
- Dosages vary depending on the condition being treated and the response to the medication—may be as high as a total of 12 grams (12,000 mg) daily or as low as 1.5 grams (1,500 mg) daily.
- Take at even intervals.
- Take each dose with a full glass of water.
- Take after meals to minimize stomach discomfort.
- Separate sulfasalazine from vitamin or mineral supplements by at least 2 hours.
- Shake suspension well before measuring dose.

Precautions:
Do not use if:
- you are allergic to sulfasalazine, sulfa, or sulfonamides.
- medicine is beyond the expiration date.

Talk to your doctor if:
- you are taking digoxin, folic acid (folate), an anti-coagulant (such as warfarin), an oral diabetes medication (such as glyburide or glipizide), phenytoin, or methotrexate.
- you have kidney disease.

Side Effects:
Major:
- rash or hives
- persistent vomiting or diarrhea
- difficulty breathing

Minor:
- nausea, vomiting, or diarrhea
- loss of appetite

Time Required for Drug to Take Effect:
Begins to take effect in 1 to 2 days.

Symptoms of Overdose:
- nausea and vomiting
- fever
- dizziness
- headache
- unconsciousness

Special Notes:
- Taking the medication on a full stomach or switching to enteric-coated tablets may minimize stomach upset, nausea, vomiting, and loss of appetite.
- Do not discontinue this medication without your doctor's consent, even if symptoms disappear.
- Sulfasalazine may turn urine and skin orange.

tacrine

Brand Name: Cognex (Parke-Davis)

Generic Available: no

Type of Drug: central nervous system drug

Used for: Treatment of dementia associated with Alzheimer disease.

How This Medication Works: Increases amount of the neurotransmitter acetylcholine in the brain.

Dosage Form and Strength: capsules (10 mg, 20 mg, 30 mg, 40 mg)

Storage:
- room temperature
- tightly closed
- protected from humidity

Administration:
- Usually taken 4 times daily.
- It is best to take on an empty stomach, but food may reduce stomach upset. Be consistent: always with food or always on an empty stomach.

Precautions:
Do not use if:
- you have had an allergic reaction to tacrine.

Talk to your doctor if:
- you take cimetidine.
- you smoke tobacco.
- you have asthma, heart problems, liver disease, seizures, stomach ulcers, or difficulty urinating.

Side Effects:

Major:
- nausea or vomiting
- diarrhea
- loss of appetite
- clumsiness

Minor:
- stomach cramping
- headache
- dizziness

Time Required for Drug to Take Effect: May
be several days to weeks before medication starts to work.

Symptoms of Overdose:
- severe nausea and vomiting
- severe muscle weakness
- sweating
- seizures
- large pupils
- irregular breathing

Special Notes:
- Your physician will obtain blood work for 16 weeks to monitor your liver function.

tamoxifen

Brand Name: Nolvadex (Zeneca)

Generic Available: no

Type of Drug: antineoplastic

Used for: Prevention of recurrence of breast cancer and treatment of advanced breast cancer.

How This Medication Works: Mechanism is not completely understood but may interfere with estrogen.

Dosage Form and Strength: tablets (10 mg, 20 mg)

Storage:
- room temperature
- tightly closed
- protected from light

Administration:
- Usual dose is 10 to 20 mg twice daily in the morning and evening.

Precautions:
Do not use if:
- you are allergic to tamoxifen.

Talk to your doctor if:
- you have cataracts, low white blood cell count (leukopenia), or low platelet level (thrombocytopenia).
- you are taking any other medication, especially antacids, cimetidine, famotidine, nizatidine, ranitidine, estrogens, or birth control pills.

Side Effects:
Major:
- confusion
- pain and swelling in legs
- shortness of breath
- vaginal bleeding

Minor:
- changes in menstruation
- bone pain
- genital itching, skin rash, or dryness
- headache
- hot flashes
- nausea and vomiting
- weight gain

Time Required for Drug to Take Effect:
Begins to have effect in 1 to 3 months but may require several more months to work.

Symptoms of Overdose:
- cataracts
- fever and chills
- low white blood cell count
- persistent sore throat

Special Notes:
- If you are still menstruating, you should use non-hormonal birth control to prevent pregnancy.
- Notify your doctor immediately if you become or think you are pregnant.

temazepam

Brand Name: Restoril (Sandoz)

Generic Available: yes

Type of Drug: sedative

Used for: Treatment of insomnia.

How This Medication Works: Enhances the
activity of the neurotransmitter gamma amino butyric
acid to depress the central nervous system.

Dosage Form and Strength: capsules (15 mg,
30 mg)

Storage:
- room temperature
- tightly closed

Administration:
- Usually taken once daily at bedtime.
- Take approximately ½ hour before the time you
  want to fall asleep.

Precautions:
Do not use if:
- you have had an allergic reaction to temazepam
  or other drugs in the benzodiazepine family such
  as diazepam, lorazepam, or oxazepam.

Talk to your doctor if:
- you are taking other medications that can depress
  the central nervous system such as alcohol, phenobarbital, or narcotics (such as codeine).
- you have asthma, other lung problems, kidney
  disease, or liver disease.
- you have been told that you snore.
- you feel you need to take for more than 7 days.

Side Effects:
Major:
- confusion or hallucinations
- seizures
- rash

Minor:
- unsteadiness or drowsiness
- slurred speech or blurred vision

Time Required for Drug to Take Effect: Starts
to have an effect within 15 to 45 minutes.

Symptoms of Overdose:
- continuing confusion or slurred speech
- severe weakness or drowsiness
- shortness of breath

Special Notes:
- Do not discontinue without your doctor's consent.
- Medication may cause a hangover effect the next day, with daytime drowsiness or sedation.
- Do not drink alcohol while taking this medication.
- The use of temazepam should be limited to 7 to 10 days to prevent worsening severity of insomnia upon discontinuation.

terfenadine

Brand Name: Seldane (Marion Merrell Dow)

Generic Available: no

Type of Drug: antihistamine

Used for: Treatment of allergies, hay fever, and hives.

How This Medication Works: Blocks histamine—a substance that causes sneezing, itching, and runny nose.

Dosage Form and Strength: tablets (60 mg)

Storage:
- room temperature
- protected from humidity

Administration:
- Take with full glass of water. Drink plenty of fluids while taking terfenadine.
- Do not exceed the dose specified by your prescription.
- Take with food if stomach upset occurs.

Precautions:
Do not use if:
- you are allergic to terfenadine or other antihistamines such as astemizole or diphenhydramine.
- you are taking erythromycin, ketoconazole, or itraconazole.
- you have severe liver disease.

Talk to your doctor if:
- you have asthma, difficulty breathing, liver disease, heart disease, high blood pressure (hypertension), or an abnormal or irregular heartbeat.
- you are taking any other medications, especially anti-infectives (such as ketoconazole, fluconazole, itraconazole, miconazole, metronidazole, or erythromycin), carbamazepine, and antidepressants.

Side Effects:
Major:
- skin rash, hives, or itching
- irregular heartbeat
- swelling of the mouth, lips, or face
- difficulty breathing
- yellowing of skin or eyes (jaundice)

Minor:
- hair loss
- cough
- menstrual disorders
- depression
- nightmares

Time Required for Drug to Take Effect: Starts to work within 1 to 2 hours.

Symptoms of Overdose:
- irregular heartbeat
- seizures or convulsions
- drowsiness or dizziness
- dryness of mouth or throat
- difficulty breathing
- trouble sleeping

Special Notes:
- Although terfenadine is considered non-sedating, there is a chance that drowsiness or dizziness may occur. Use caution when operating a motor vehicle or dangerous machinery.
- Check with your physician or pharmacist before you use any over-the-counter medications.
- Tell the doctor you are taking terfenadine before you have a skin test for allergies.
- Do not drink alcohol or take other medications that cause drowsiness or mental slowing.
- If you experience dryness of the mouth, try sugar-less candy or gum, ice chips, or a saliva substitute.
- Tell the doctor or dentist you are taking terfenadine if you are going to have surgery or emergency treatment.

theophylline

Brand Names:

Theobid Jr. Duratuss (Russ)
Theobid Duracaps (Russ)
Theoclear L.A. (Central)
Theo-Dur (Key)
Theolair (3M)
Theolair-SR (3M)
Theo-Sav (Savage)
Theospan-SR (Laser)
Theo–24 (Whitby)
Theovent (Schering)
Theox (Carnrick)
T-Phyl (Purdue-Frederick)
Uniphyl (Purdue-Frederick)
Aerolate (Fleming)
Bronkodyl (Winthrop)
Constant-T (Ciba-Geigy)
Elixophyllin (Forest)
Elixophyllin SR (Forest)
Quibron-T/SR Dividose (Bristol-Meyers Squibb)
Quibron-T Dividose (Bristol-Meyers Squibb)
Respbid (Boehringer Ingelheim)
Slo-Phyllin (Rhone-Poulenc Rorer)
Slo-Phyllin Gyrocaps (Rhone-Poulenc Rorer)
Slo-bid Gyrocaps (Rhone-Poulenc Rorer)
Sustaire (Pfizer)

Generic Available: yes

Type of Drug: bronchodilator

Used for: Treatment of asthma, chronic bronchitis, and emphysema.

How This Medication Works: Causes the passageways in the lungs to dilate and strengthens the diaphragm muscle to help in breathing.

Dosage Form and Strength:

- tablets (100 mg, 125 mg, 200 mg, 250 mg, 300 mg, 400 mg, 450 mg, 500 mg)

- capsules (50 mg, 60 mg, 65 mg, 75 mg, 100 mg, 125 mg, 130 mg, 200 mg, 250 mg, 260 mg, 300 mg)

Storage:
- room temperature
- protected from humidity

Administration:
- Swallow tablets and capsules whole; do not crush or chew.
- Certain theophylline products need to be taken on an empty stomach, while others work better or cause less stomach upset when taken with food. Make sure to ask your doctor and pharmacist how to take your theophylline: with or without food or with a full glass of water on an empty stomach.
- This medication is used to prevent breathing problems. It must be taken on a continuous basis to ensure adequate concentrations in the bloodstream.

Precautions:
Do not use if:
- you have had an allergic reaction to theophylline or other xanthine-related substances such as caffeine.

Talk to your doctor if:
- you have fever, liver disease, respiratory infections, diarrhea, enlarged prostate, heart disease, high blood pressure (hypertension), ulcers, heartburn, other stomach problems, breast disease, or thyroid disease.

- you are taking any other medications, especially steroids, antibiotics, nicotine replacement products, or medications for heart disease, high blood pressure, stomach problems, or seizures.

Side Effects:

Major:
- skin rash, hives, or itching
- bloody or black, tarry stools
- dizziness or light-headedness
- difficulty breathing
- irregular heartbeat
- headache
- increased urination
- loss of appetite
- trembling or muscle twitching
- nausea, vomiting, diarrhea, or stomach cramps
- irritability or trouble sleeping
- seizures or convulsions

Minor:
- nausea
- nervousness
- tremor

Time Required for Drug to Take Effect: Starts to work in 1½ to 3 hours, but you must take theophylline on a continuous basis.

Symptoms of Overdose:
- dizziness or light-headedness
- difficulty breathing
- irregular heartbeat
- headache
- increased urination

- irritability
- loss of appetite
- trembling or muscle twitching
- nausea, vomiting, diarrhea, or stomach cramps
- seizures or convulsions

Special Notes:

- Check with your physician or pharmacist before using any over-the-counter medications.
- Theophylline has caffeinelike activities. Therefore, avoid consuming large amounts of caffeine.
- You will need to have blood tests while you are taking theophylline to determine how much is in your bloodstream.
- Certain medications, cigarette smoking, and eating charcoal-broiled foods can increase your liver's ability to metabolize theophylline. Discuss any new medications, cigarette smoking, and your diet with your doctor or pharmacist.

thioridazine

Brand Name: Mellaril (Sandoz)

Generic Available: yes

Type of Drug: antipsychotic

Used for: Treatment of psychotic disorders (schizophrenia) and acute agitation (symptoms of dementia-like hallucinations, suspiciousness, or hostility).

How This Medication Works: Blocks the neurotransmitter dopamine in the central nervous system.

Dosage Form and Strength:
- tablets (10 mg, 15 mg, 25 mg, 50 mg, 100 mg, 150 mg, 200 mg)
- oral solution (30 mg/mL, 100 mg/mL)

Storage:
- room temperature
- tightly closed

Administration:
- Usually taken 3 times daily.
- Dilute oral solution in water or juice.
- Shake suspension well before use.

Precautions:
Do not use if:
- you have had an allergic reaction to thioridazine, chlorpromazine, perphenazine, or other medications from the phenothiazine family.
- you have Parkinson disease.

Talk to your doctor if:
- you are taking any other medications, especially antacids, antidiarrheals, phenobarbital, carbamazepine, lithium, meperidine, propranolol, or tricyclic antidepressants (such as amitriptyline).
- you have liver disease, stomach ulcers, seizures, heart disease, or enlarged prostate.

Side Effects:
Major:
- blurred vision
- skin rash or sunburn
- problems speaking or swallowing
- lip smacking or restlessness

Minor:
- constipation
- dizziness
- drowsiness
- dry mouth

Time Required for Drug to Take Effect: May take several weeks before desired effect is seen.

Symptoms of Overdose:
- drowsiness
- difficulty arousing
- agitation
- restlessness
- seizures
- fever

Special Notes:
- Use a sunblock with at least SPF 15 when outside because thioridazine may increase your sensitivity to the sun.
- If you experience dryness of the mouth, try sugarless candy or gum, ice chips, or a saliva substitute.
- If using antacids, separate doses of thioridazine and antacid by 2 hours.
- Do not discontinue without first talking with your doctor.
- Check with your physician or pharmacist before using any over-the-counter medications.
- Thioridazine may cause movement disorders; tell your doctor about any involuntary muscle movements or spasms.
- Do not allow oral solution to come in contact with skin.

thiothixene

Brand Name: Navane (Roerig)

Generic Available: yes

Type of Drug: antipsychotic

Used for: Treatment of psychotic disorders such as schizophrenia.

How This Medication Works: Blocks a chemical messenger receptor in the central nervous system.

Dosage Form and Strength:
- capsules (1 mg, 2 mg, 5 mg, 10 mg, 20 mg)
- oral concentrate (5 mg/mL)

Storage:
- room temperature
- tightly closed

Administration:
- Usually taken 2 to 3 times daily.
- May be taken with food to reduce stomach irritation.
- Dilute oral concentrate in half a tall glass of water, soda, or juice before taking.
- If using antacids, separate doses of thiothixene and antacids by 2 hours.

Precautions:
Do not use if:
- you have had an allergic reaction to thiothixene or chlorprothixene.
- you have Parkinson disease.

Talk to your doctor if:
- you are taking any other medications, especially antacids, antidiarrheals, phenobarbital, carbamazepine, lithium, meperidine, propranolol, or tricyclic antidepressants (such as amitriptyline or imipramine).
- you have liver disease, stomach ulcers, seizures, heart disease, urination problems, or enlarged prostate.

Side Effects:
Major:
- blurred vision
- skin rash or sunburn
- problems speaking or swallowing
- lip smacking or restlessness

Minor:
- constipation
- dizziness or drowsiness
- dry mouth

Time Required for Drug to Take Effect: May take several weeks before desired effect is seen.

Symptoms of Overdose:
- severe drowsiness
- agitation or restlessness
- seizures
- fever

Special Notes:
- Use a sunblock with at least SPF 15 when outside because thiothixene may increase your sensitivity to the sun.

- If you experience dryness of the mouth, try sugarless candy or gum, ice chips, or a saliva substitute.
- Do not discontinue without first talking with your doctor.
- Check with your physician or pharmacist before using any over-the-counter medications.
- Thiothixene may cause movement disorders; tell your doctor about any involuntary muscle movements or spasms.
- Do not allow oral concentrate to come in contact with skin.

thyroid hormone (desiccated)

Brand Name: none

Generic Available: yes

Type of Drug: hormone

Used for: Treatment of low levels of thyroid hormone (hypothyroidism).

How This Medication Works: Increases thyroid hormone levels to healthy range.

Dosage Form and Strength: tablets (15 mg, 30 mg, 60 mg, 90 mg, 120 mg, 180 mg, 240 mg, 300 mg)

Storage:
- room temperature
- tightly closed
- protected from light

Administration:

- Usual dosage is 60 mg to 120 mg once daily. The dosage will be adjusted monthly until the desired level of thyroid hormone is reached.

Precautions:

Do not use if:

- you have had an allergic reaction to thyroid hormone, levothyroxine, thyroglobulin, liothyronine, or liotrix.
- you have hyperthyroidism.

Talk to your doctor if:

- you have heart disease, diabetes, adrenocortical disease, pituitary disease, or malabsorption disease (celiac disease).
- you are taking any other medication, especially anticoagulants (such as warfarin), diabetes medications (such as insulin, glipizide, glyburide, or tolbutamide), digoxin, cholesterol medications (such as lovastatin, cholestyramine, or niacin), cough and cold medicines, seizure medications (such as phenytoin, phenobarbital, or carbamazepine), cholestyramine, or colestipol.

Side Effects:

Major:

- skin rash, hives, or itching
- changes in appetite
- chest pain
- diarrhea or vomiting
- difficulty breathing
- fast or irregular heartbeat
- hand tremor

- headache
- heat intolerance
- increased sweating
- irritability, nervousness, or trouble sleeping
- leg cramps
- weight loss

Minor:
- clumsiness or weakness
- coldness
- constipation
- dry skin
- headache
- listlessness or sleepiness
- depression
- muscle aches
- weight gain

Time Required for Drug to Take Effect:
Usually takes 1 to 2 months to reach normal thyroid levels. Most people will have to take thyroid medication for life.

Symptoms of Overdose:
- chest pain
- diarrhea or vomiting
- difficulty breathing
- fast or irregular heartbeat
- hand tremor
- headache
- heat intolerance
- increased sweating
- irritability, nervousness, or trouble sleeping
- weight loss

Special Notes:
- Thyroid medications are often started with low doses and increased slowly to avoid nervousness, chest pain, and increased heart rate.
- Do not discontinue without your doctor's consent.

ticlopidine

Brand Name: Ticlid (Roche)

Generic Available: no

Type of Drug: blood modifier

Used for: Prevention of strokes caused by blood clots in the brain.

How This Medication Works: Decreases platelet stickiness to discourage clots.

Dosage Form and Strength: tablets (250 mg)

Storage:
- room temperature
- tightly closed
- protected from light

Administration:
- Usually taken twice daily with food.
- If you miss a dose, you can take the dose as soon as you remember. If it is time for the next dose, skip the missed dose and return to the regular schedule; do not double the dose.
- If using antacids, separate doses of ticlopidine and antacid by 2 hours.

Precautions:

Do not use if:
- you have had an allergic reaction to ticlopidine.
- you have bleeding, hemophilia, low platelet levels, low white blood cell count (leukopenia), or severe liver disease.

Talk to your doctor if:
- you have kidney disease or stomach ulcers.
- you have recently had surgery or been injured.
- you are taking any other medications, especially anticoagulants (such as heparin or warfarin), aspirin, nonsteroidal anti-inflammatory agents (such as ibuprofen, indomethacin, or naproxen), salicylates, or antacids.

Side Effects:

Major:
- bleeding (see signs of overdose)
- fever and chills
- ringing in the ears (tinnitus)
- skin rash
- skin yellowing (jaundice)
- frequent or persistent sore throats
- white spots in the mouth

Minor:
- nausea or vomiting
- diarrhea
- dizziness
- headache
- stomach irritation and cramps

Time Required for Drug to Take Effect: Starts
to work in 1 to 2 weeks.

Symptoms of Overdose:
- severe back pain
- bleeding gums
- black, tarry stool or red blood in your stools
- unusual, frequent, or severe bruising
- coughing up blood
- cuts or wounds that won't stop bleeding
- decreased alertness
- dizziness
- blood in eyes
- severe or persistent headache
- joint pain or swelling
- menstrual bleeding (heavy or unexpected)
- nose bleeds
- paralysis
- speech difficulty
- stomach pain or bloating
- bloody, pink, or red urine
- unusual tiredness or weakness
- unsteadiness on you feet

Special Notes:
- Regular blood tests are necessary to make sure you do not develop side effects.
- Tell your doctor or dentist you are taking ticlopidine if you are going to have surgery, a tooth extraction, or emergency treatment; ticlopidine therapy is usually stopped for 10 to 14 days before surgery.
- Tell your doctor if you have had any falls while taking this medication because there is a risk of internal bleeding.

timolol

Brand Name: Timoptic (Merck)

Generic Available: no

Type of Drug: topical ophthalmologic agent

Used for: Treatment of glaucoma.

How This Medication Works: Exact mechanism is unknown, but it appears to lower the pressure in the eye by decreasing fluid production and possibly encouraging fluid outflow.

Dosage Form and Strength: ophthalmic solution (0.25%, 0.5%)

Storage:
- room temperature
- tightly closed
- protected from light

Administration:
- Usually administered in both eyes once or twice daily.
- Wash your hands thoroughly with soap and water before using.
- Avoid touching the dropper tip of bottle against your eye or anything else.
- While tilting your head back, pull down the lower eyelid with your index finger to form a pocket.
- With the other hand, hold the bottle (tip down) as close to the eye as possible without touching it.

- Brace the remaining fingers of that hand against your face.
- Gently squeeze the dropper so that one drop falls into the pocket made by the lower eyelid.
- Close your eye gently and avoid blinking.
- Replace and tighten the cap right away and do not wipe or rinse the dropper tip.
- Wash your hands to remove any medication.
- The eye can hold only one drop at a time; wait at least 5 minutes between each drop if you have more than one drop to apply.

Precautions:

Do not use if:

- you have had an allergic reaction to timolol or other beta blockers such as acebutolol, atenolol, betaxolol, carteolol, labetalol, metoprolol, nadolol, oxprenolol, penbutolol, pindolol, propranolol, or sotalol.
- you have asthma, lung disease, heart failure, heart block, cardiac shock, or slow heart rate.

Talk to your doctor if:

- you have experienced heart failure.
- you have breathing problems, cerebrovascular insufficiency, a history of heart block, diabetes, an overactive thyroid (hyperthyroidism), myasthenia gravis, or peripheral vascular disease.
- you are taking any other medication, especially beta blockers (such as acebutolol, atenolol, betaxolol, carteolol, labetalol, metoprolol, nadolol, oxprenolol, penbutolol, pindolol, propranolol, or sotalol) and asthma or breathing medications (such as inhalers or theophylline).

Side Effects:
Major:
- severe irritation, redness, or swelling of eye or eyelid
- skin rash, hives, or itching
- wheezing or trouble breathing
- anxiety
- chest pain
- confusion
- depression
- swelling of feet, ankles, or lower legs
- slow heartbeat
- trouble sleeping
- hallucinations
- headache
- unusual tiredness
- weakness
- nausea, vomiting, or stomach pain
- dizziness

Minor:
- stinging of the eye upon administration that should stop in a few minutes.

Time Required for Drug to Take Effect:
Begins to work immediately and improves glaucoma only as long as it is continued.

Symptoms of Overdose:
- heart failure
- slow heartrate
- heart block
- wheezing or trouble breathing
- low blood pressure

Special Notes:
- Eye drops are hard to use; have someone help you put them in if possible. Tell your doctor if you cannot put them in yourself and have no one to help you.
- Tell the doctor or dentist you are taking timolol if you are going to have surgery or emergency treatment.
- Timolol may cause light sensitivity; use sunglasses.

tramadol

Brand Name: Ultram (Robins)

Generic Available: no

Type of Drug: analgesic

Used for: Relief of pain.

How This Medication Works: Alters the perception of pain in the central nervous system.

Dosage Form and Strength: tablets (50 mg)

Storage:
- room temperature
- protected from humidity

Administration:
- Take with milk or food if stomach upset occurs.
- Do not exceed the maximum number of doses per day. Never take more tablets per dose, than your doctor has prescribed.

Precautions:
Do not use if:
- you are allergic to tramadol.

Talk to your doctor if:
- you have substance abuse problems or alcoholism; brain disease or head injury; colitis; seizures; emotional problems or mental illness; emphysema, asthma, or other lung diseases; kidney, liver, or thyroid disease; prostate problems or problems with urination; or gallbladder disease or gallstones.
- you are taking any other medications, especially naltrexone and medications that can cause drowsiness such as antihistamines, barbiturates (phenobarbital), benzodiazepines (diazepam, alprazolam, lorazepam), muscle relaxants, or antidepressants.

Side Effects:
Major:
- skin rash or hives
- irregular breathing or difficulty breathing
- seizures
- painful or difficult urination
- frequent urge to urinate
- fast, slow, or pounding heartbeat
- hallucinations or severe confusion
- depression
- trembling or uncontrolled muscle movements

Minor:
- constipation
- drowsiness
- dry mouth

- general feeling of discomfort or illness
- loss of appetite
- difficulty sleeping
- nervousness or restlessness

Time Required for Drug to Take Effect: Starts to work within 30 to 60 minutes.

Symptoms of Overdose:

- cold, clammy skin
- seizures
- diarrhea
- severe dizziness, drowsiness, or confusion
- continued nausea or vomiting
- severe nervousness or restlessness
- difficulty breathing
- slowed heartbeat

Special Notes:

- This medication may make you drowsy or dizzy. Do not operate a motor vehicle or other machinery while you are taking this medication.
- Tramadol will cause constipation. This side effect may be diminished by drinking 6 to 8 full glasses of water each day. Increase fresh fruit in your diet. If using tramadol for chronic pain, ask you doctor about a stool softener–laxative combination.
- Check with your physician or pharmacist before using any over-the-counter medications.
- It is not known whether tramadol may be habit-forming (mental or physical dependence). Therefore, it is important to report any cravings to your doctor or pharmacist.
- Do not stop taking this medication abruptly.

- Nausea and vomiting may occur after the first few doses; this effect should diminish with time.
- Do not drink alcohol while taking this medication.
- If you experience dry mouth, try sugarless candy or gum, ice chips, or a saliva substitute.
- If you think you or anyone else may have taken an overdose, get emergency help immediately.
- Use this medication as prescribed; do not exceed the dose or frequency prescribed by your doctor.

trazodone

Brand Name: Desyrel (Mead Johnson)

Generic Available: yes

Type of Drug: antidepressant

Used for: Treatment of depression, anxiety, and sleep problems associated with depression.

How This Medication Works: Increases the action of serotonin and other neurotransmitters in the brain.

Dosage Form and Strength: tablets (50 mg, 100 mg, 150 mg, 300 mg)

Storage:
- room temperature
- tightly closed

Administration:
- Initial dose given once daily at bedtime for older adults, but may be increased to 2 to 3 times daily.

- May be taken with food to reduce stomach upset.

Precautions:

Do not use if:
- you have ever had an allergic reaction to trazodone.

Talk to your doctor if:
- you have heart disease.
- you have ever had liver or kidney problems.
- you are taking medication for high blood pressure (hypertension), depression, anxiety, sleep disorders, or any mental problem.

Side Effects:

Major:
- confusion, agitation, or extreme excitement
- dizziness or fainting when standing up
- chest pain
- shortness of breath
- rapid heartbeat or unusually slow heartbeat
- prolonged painful penile erection

Minor:
- drowsiness
- vivid dreams
- dizziness
- dry mouth
- headache
- nausea or vomiting
- unpleasant taste
- blurred vision
- constipation
- muscle aches or pains
- unusual fatigue or weakness

Time Required for Drug to Take Effect: May
start to improve some symptoms within the first few
weeks, but the full benefit may take from 4 to 8 weeks.

Symptoms of Overdose:
- severe drowsiness
- weakness
- severe nausea or vomiting
- dizziness or fainting when standing up
- headache
- shivering

Special Notes:
- Know which "target symptoms" (restlessness,
  worry, fear, or changes in sleep or appetite) you
  are being treated for and be prepared to tell your
  doctor if your target symptoms are improving,
  worsening, or unchanged.
- Do not drink alcohol when using this medicine.
- Never increase your dose without the advice of
  your doctor.
- Do not discontinue without first talking with your
  doctor.

triamcinolone (topical)

Brand Names:
Aristocort (Fujisawa)
Kenalog (Westwood-Squibb)

Generic Available: yes

Type of Drug: general topical

Used for: Treatment of dermatitis, eczema, psoriasis, poison ivy, and other skin disorders.

How This Medication Works: Relieves skin inflammation, redness, swelling, itching, and discomfort.

Dosage Form and Strength:

- aerosol (0.015%)
- cream (0.025%, 0.1%, 0.5%)
- lotion (0.025%, 0.1%)
- ointment (0.025%, 0.1%, 0.5%)

Storage:

- room temperature
- tightly closed
- protected from light

Administration:

- Clean affected area with soap and water, pat the area almost dry with a clean towel (skin should be slightly moist).
- Apply a thin layer to affected area twice daily or as directed.
- Do not bandage or cover unless directed by your doctor.
- Do not apply on cuts or open wounds.
- If you miss a dose of triamcinolone, apply the dose as soon as you remember. If it is near the time for your next dose, skip the dose and return to the usual schedule; do not apply double the dose.
- If you are using the lotion or aerosol, shake well before each application.

Precautions:

Do not use if:
- you have had an allergic reaction to triamcinolone, amcinonide, betamethasone, clocortolone, cortisone, desonide, desoximetasone,
dexamethasone, diflorasone, flumethasone, ffluo-
cinonide, fluorometholone, fluorometholone, flurandrenolide, halcinonide, hydrocortisone,
methylprednisolone, prednisolone, prednisone,
triamcinolone, or any other steroid.

Talk to your doctor if:
- you have blood vessel disease (vascular disease),
cataracts, diabetes, fungal infections, glaucoma,
shingles, stomach ulcers, skin infections, or tuberculosis.

Side Effects:

Major:
- blistering
- bruising
- increased hair growth
- infection
- irritation
- loss of skin color

Minor:
- acne
- burning or stinging
- dryness
- itching
- redness

Time Required for Drug to Take Effect:
Begins to improve symptoms after 1 week.

Symptoms of Overdose: Usually not a problem when used on the skin. If accidentally taken orally, contact your doctor or a poison center for instructions.

Special Notes:
- Do not use for infections other than the one for which it was prescribed.
- Do not use around the eyes.
- Keep the affected area clean and dry, wear freshly laundered clothing, and avoid tight-fitting clothing.
- If you do not get improvement or the condition gets worse after 1 week, call your doctor.

triamcinolone acetonide (inhaler)

Brand Name: Azmacort (Rhone-Poulenc Rorer)

Generic Available: no

Type of Drug: respiratory (antiasthma, antiallergic)

Used for: Prevention of allergy and asthma attacks.

How This Medication Works: Prevents the lungs from reacting to allergens and causing an asthma attack.

Dosage Form and Strength: inhaler (100 µg/inhalation)

Storage:
- room temperature
- protected from humidity

Administration:

- This medication is used to prevent asthma attacks. It is not useful once an acute asthma attack has begun. In fact, it may make the attack worse. Therefore, it is important to take this on a continuous basis, even when you are not having symptoms, to prevent them from occurring.
- Have your doctor or pharmacist demonstrate the proper procedure for using and practice your technique in front of them.
- If you have more than one inhaler, it is important to administer your inhalers in the correct order. If you are using triamcinolone and another inhaler, use the other inhaler first. Wait at least 5 minutes before inhaling triamcinolone after you have used the first medication. If you are using all 3 classes of inhalers, use the triamcinolone inhaler last.

Precautions:

Do not use if:
- you are allergic to triamcinolone or steroids such as beclomethasone, prednisone, dexamethasone, or flunisolide.

Talk to your doctor if:
- you have lung disease, any type of infection (especially of the throat, mouth, or lungs, including tuberculosis), bone disease, diabetes, problems with your digestive tract (such as ulcers, colitis, or diverticulitis), eye disease (including glaucoma), heart disease, high blood pressure (hypertension), high blood cholesterol levels, kidney disease, liver disease, myasthenia gravis, or thyroid disease.

- you have had a recent heart attack.
- you are taking any other medications, especially medication for diabetes.

Side Effects:

Major:
- skin rash, hives, or itching
- difficulty breathing
- signs or symptoms of infections
- creamy white, cottage cheese-like patches inside the mouth
- irregular heartbeat
- nausea or vomiting
- decreased or blurred vision
- difficulty swallowing
- increased blood pressure
- increased thirst
- depression or mood changes
- swelling of face, feet, or lower legs
- unusual weight gain
- bloody or black, tarry stools
- back or rib pain

Minor:
- acne or other skin problems
- fullness or rounding out of the face
- menstrual problems
- muscle weakness, cramps, or pain
- upset stomach, bloated feeling, or gas
- diarrhea or constipation
- cough without other signs of infection
- dizziness or light-headedness
- headache
- heartburn or indigestion

- hoarseness or other voice changes
- loss of appetite
- loss of smell or taste
- nervousness
- unpleasant taste
- dry, irritated mouth, tongue, or throat
- general discomfort, illness, shakiness, or faintness
- increasd appetite
- increased sweating
- trouble sleeping

Time Required for Drug to Take Effect: Starts
to work within minutes. However, it takes anywhere
from 1 to 4 weeks to receive enough medication to
prevent an asthma attack.

Symptoms of Overdose:
- difficulty breathing
- irregular heartbeat
- nausea or vomiting
- decreased or blurred vision
- difficulty swallowing
- severely increased thirst
- depression or mood changes
- swelling of face, feet, or lower legs

Special Notes:
- Check with your physician or pharmacist before
  you use any over-the-counter medications.
- Be sure that you keep track of how many inhalations are left and get your medication refilled
  about 1 week before you expect to run out.
- Clean your inhaler every day. Your doctor or pharmacist will show you how.

- Sometimes a spacer device is used with your inhaler. A spacer device helps the medication get to the lungs instead of staying in the mouth or throat.
- Gargle and rinse your mouth out after each use to prevent hoarseness, throat irritation, and infections in the mouth. Do not swallow the solution you use to rinse with because it may contain some left-over medication which can get into your bloodstream.
- Tell the doctor or dentist that you are taking triamcinolone before you have any kind of surgery or emergency treatment. It may be helpful to wear an ID bracelet.

triamterene and hydrochlorothiazide combination

Brand Names:
Dyazide (SK Beecham)
Maxzide (Lederle)

Generic Available: yes

Type of Drug: diuretic

Used for: Treatment of fluid retention (edema) and high blood pressure (hypertension).

How This Medication Works: Interferes with sodium reabsorption in the kidney, thereby increasing water excretion. Triamterene is used in combination with hydrochlorothiazide to prevent the loss of potassium.

Dosage Form and Strength:
- tablets (37.5 mg triamterene/25 mg hydrochlorothiazide, 75 mg/50 mg)
- capsules (37.5 mg/25 mg, 50 mg/25 mg)

Storage:
- room temperature
- tightly closed
- protected from humidity

Administration:
- Usually taken once daily, in the morning.
- May be taken without regard to meals; take with
  food or milk if stomach upset occurs.

Precautions:
Do not use if:
- you are allergic to hydrochlorothiazide or other
  thiazide diuretics such as chlorthalidone or metolazone.
- you are allergic to triamterene.
- you are allergic to sulfa drugs, including diabetes
  medication (tolazamide, glipizide, or glyburide),
  acetazolamide, loop diuretics (such as furosemide
  or bumetanide), or sulfa antibacterial medication
  (such as sulfamethoxazole).

Talk to your doctor if:
- you have liver disease, kidney disease, or gout.
- you are taking allopurinol, warfarin, calcium supplements, digoxin, lithium, loop diuretics (such as
  furosemide, bumetanide, or torsemide), methyldopa, oral diabetes medication (such as tolazamide, glipizide, or glyburide), insulin, vitamin D,
  cholestyramine, nonsteroidal anti-inflammatory

drugs (such as ibuprofen, sulindac, indomethacin, or diclofenac), a potassium supplement, amantadine, an angiotensin-convertin enzyme inhibitor (such as captopril, enalapril, lisinopril, or benazepril), or cimetidine.

Side Effects:

Major:

- seizures
- chest pain
- irregular heartbeat
- skin rash

Minor:

- dry mouth
- drowsiness
- headache
- impotence

Time Required for Drug to Take Effect: Starts
to work 2 to 4 hours after the first dose, but maximum therapeutic effect may take several days.

Symptoms of Overdose:

- nausea and vomiting
- diarrhea
- profound muscle weakness
- profound low blood pressure

Special Notes:

- Avoid salt substitutes with potassium. Triamterene may cause your body to retain potassium.
- Your doctor will check blood count, kidney function, and electrolyte (sodium and potassium) levels periodically during therapy.

- Use a sunblock with at least SPF 15 when outside because this medication may increase your sensitivity to the sun.
- If you experience dryness of the mouth, try sugarless candy or gum, ice chips, or a saliva substitute.
- Weigh yourself daily. If you gain or lose more than 1 pound per day, call your doctor.
- Changing positions slowly when sitting and/or standing up may help decrease dizziness caused by this medication.
- If you notice dizziness or drowsiness, avoid activities requiring mental alertness, such as operating a motor vehicle or dangerous machinery.
- If you have diabetes, you may need to check your blood glucose more frequently while taking this medication.

triazolam

Brand Name: Halcion (Upjohn)

Generic Available: no

Type of Drug: sedative

Used for: Treatment of insomnia.

How This Medication Works: Enhances the activity of the neurotransmitter gamma amino butyric acid to depress the central nervous system.

Dosage Form and Strength: tablets (0.125 mg, 0.25 mg)

Storage:
- room temperature
- tightly closed

Administration:
- Usually taken once daily at bedtime.
- Take approximately ½ hour before the time you want to fall asleep.

Precautions:
Do not use if:
- you have had an allergic reaction to triazolam or other drugs in the benzodiazepine family such as diazepam, lorazepam, or oxazepam.

Talk to your doctor if:
- you are taking other medications that can depress the central nervous system such as alcohol, phenobarbital, or narcotics (such as codeine).
- you have asthma, other lung problems, kidney disease, or liver disease.
- you have been told that you snore.
- you feel you need to continue this medicine for more than 7 days.

Side Effects:
Major:
- confusion or hallucinations
- seizures
- rash
- difficulty concentrating

Minor:
- unsteadiness
- drowsiness or slurred speech
- blurred vision

Time Required for Drug to Take Effect: Starts
to have an effect within 15 to 45 minutes.

Symptoms of Overdose:
- continuing or worsening confusion or slurred speech
- severe weakness or drowsiness
- shortness of breath

Special Notes:
- Do not discontinue without your doctor's consent.
- Medication may cause a hangover effect the next day, with daytime drowsiness or sedation.
- Do not drink alcohol while taking this medication.
- The use of triazolam should be limited to 7 to 10 days to prevent worsening severity of insomnia on discontinuation.

trifluoperazine

Brand Name: Stelazine (SK Beecham)

Generic Available: yes

Type of Drug: antipsychotic

Used for: Treatment of psychotic disorders (schizophrenia).

How This Medication Works: Blocks neurotransmitters in the central nervous system.

Dosage Form and Strength:
- tablets (1 mg, 2 mg, 5 mg, 10 mg)
- oral solution (10 mg/mL)

Storage:
- room temperature
- tightly closed

Administration:
- Usually taken twice daily.
- Oral solution may be diluted in a beverage such as water or soda.
- May be taken with food to reduce stomach irritation.
- If taking over-the-counter antacids wait 1 to 2 hours between taking antacid and trifluoperazine.

Precautions:
Do not use if:
- you have had an allergic reaction to trifluoperazine or other drugs in the phenothiazine family such as chlorpromazine or thioridazine.

Talk to your doctor if:
- you are taking any other medications, especially antacids, antidiarrheals, phenobarbital, carbamazepine, lithium, meperidine, propranolol, and tricyclic antidepressants (such as amitriptyline or imipramine).
- you have liver disease, stomach ulcers, seizures, heart disease, or enlarged prostate.

Side Effects:
Major:
- blurred vision
- skin rash or sunburn
- problems speaking or swallowing
- lip smacking
- restlessness

Minor:
- constipation
- dizziness or drowsiness
- dry mouth

Time Required for Drug to Take Effect: Takes several weeks before desired effect is seen.

Symptoms of Overdose:
- severe drowsiness
- agitation or restlessness
- seizures
- fever

Special Notes:
- Do not drink alcohol while taking this medication.
- Do not discontinue without your doctor's consent.
- Trifluoperazine may cause movement disorders. Tell your doctor about any involuntary muscle movements or spasms.
- Do not allow oral solution to touch skin.
- Use a sunblock with at least SPF 15 when outside because trifluoperazine may increase your sensitivity to the sun.

trihexyphenidyl

Brand Names:
Artane (Lederle)
Artane Sequels (Lederle)

Generic Available: yes

Type of Drug: antiparkinsonian (anticholinergic)

Used for: Treatment of Parkinson disease and parkonsonism.

How This Medication Works: Blocks the action of the neurotransmitter acetylcholine, restoring the balance between it and the neurotransmitter dopamine.

Dosage Form and Strength:
- tablets (2 mg, 5 mg)
- sustained-release capsules (5 mg)
- liquid/elixir (2 mg/5 mL)

Storage:
- room temperature
- tightly closed

Administration:
- Regular tablets usually taken 2 to 3 times daily.
- Elixir usually taken 2 to 3 times daily.
- Sustained-release capsules usually taken once or twice daily (12 hours apart).
- May take with food if stomach upset occurs.

Precautions:
Do not use if:
- you have ever had an allergic reaction to trihexyphenidyl.
- you have narrow angle glaucoma (angle closure type), colitis, severe constipation, prostate problems, myasthenia gravis, or tardive dyskinesia.

Talk to your doctor if:
- you are taking medicines for anxiety, depression, sleep problems, hallucinations, or other mental conditions.

- you have dry mouth, constipation, urinary retention, breathing problems, liver disease, kidney
  disease, or rapid heartbeat.
- you are using medicines for dizziness, seasickness, upset stomach, cramping (muscle relaxants),
  hiatal hernia, allergies, irregular heartbeat, or pain.
- you are taking metoclopramide or antipsychotics
  such as haloperidol and thioridazine.

Side Effects:
Major:
- eye pain
- dilated pupils
- severe constipation
- difficult urination
- painful urination
- seizures
- severe agitation
- severe confusion
- hot, dry, flushed skin
- fever
- numbness in the fingers
- severe muscle weakness or cramping

Minor:
- dizziness
- drowsiness
- sedation
- dry mouth
- blurred vision
- mild constipation

Time Required for Drug to Take Effect: Relief
of symptoms occurs within 1 to 2 hours.

Symptoms of Overdose:
- eye pain and dilated pupils
- severe constipation
- seizures
- severe confusion, agitation, or psychosis
- hot, dry, flushed skin, fever
- severe muscle weakness or cramping
- coma, stupor

Special Notes:
- Anticholinergic drugs are usually not recommended in older adults because older adults may be more sensitive to side effects.
- Many other medicines have similar side effects. To avoid the possibility of having side effects add up, have your doctor and pharmacist check all medicines, including over-the-counter medicines.
- Do not drink alcohol when using this medicine.
- Avoid staying out in hot weather for long periods of time because this medicine may increase your risk of heat stroke.
- Do not discontinue without your doctor's consent.

valproic acid

Brand Names:
Depakote (Abbott)
Depakene (Abbott)

Depakote Sprinkle
(Abbott)

Generic Available: yes

Type of Drug: antiepileptic

Used for: Treatment of epilepsy and migraine headaches.

How This Medication Works: Believed to increase the amount of the neurotransmitter gamma amino butyric acid to prevent seizures and migraines.

Dosage Form and Strength:
- tablets (125 mg, 250 mg, 500 mg)
- capsules (125 mg)
- delayed-release capsules (125 mg)
- oral syrup (250 mg/5 mL)

Storage:
- room temperature
- tightly closed

Administration:
- swallow tablets, capsule, and delayed-release capsules whole; do not chew, crush, or break.
- take syrup alone or mix with other liquids such as water or juice.

Precautions:
Do not use if:
- you have had an allergic reaction to valproic acid.

Talk to your doctor if:
- you are taking any other medications, especially chlorpromazine, cimetidine, rifampin, salicylates (such as aspirin), benzodiazepines (such as diazepam, clonazepam, or lorazepam), carbamazepine, lamotrigine, phenytoin, phenobarbital, warfarin, or zidovudine.
- you have kidney or liver disease.

Side Effects:

Major:
- mood changes
- double vision
- unusual bleeding
- continued nausea or vomiting

Minor:
- diarrhea
- hair loss
- nausea or vomiting
- trembling of the hands
- weight loss or gain
- dizziness
- drowsiness

Time Required for Drug to Take Effect:

Decreases the number and/or frequency of seizures and migraines as long as it is continued.

Symptoms of Overdose:

- hallucinations
- sedation
- double vision or spots before the eyes
- incoordination

Special Notes:

- This medication may cause drowsiness. Use caution when operating a motor vehicle or dangerous machinery.
- Do not discontinue without first talking with your doctor.
- You will need to have periodic blood tests to monitor therapy.

venlafaxine

Brand Name: Effexor (Wyeth-Ayerst)

Generic Available: no

Type of Drug: antidepressant

Used for: Treatment of depression.

How This Medication Works: May prolong the action of the neurotransmitters serotonin and norepinephrine and block them in certain parts of the brain.

Dosage Form and Strength: tablets (25 mg, 37.5 mg, 50 mg, 75 mg, 100 mg)

Storage:
- room temperature
- tightly closed

Administration:
- Usually taken 2 or 3 times daily.
- Take with food.

Precautions:

Do not use if:
- you are allergic to venlafaxine.
- you are taking, or have taken in the past 14 days, a monoamine oxidase (MAO) inhibitor such as phenelzine or tranylcypromine.

Talk to your doctor if:
- you have ever had liver problems, kidney problems, or seizures.
- you have high blood pressure (hypertension) or take medicines to lower your blood pressure.

Side Effects:

Major:
- headache
- seizures
- dizziness or fainting when standing up
- vision changes
- chest pain
- rapid heart beat
- swollen feet or legs
- difficulty breathing
- unusual restlessness, excitement, or confusion
- severe nausea or vomiting
- severe weakness
- difficulty urinating

Minor:
- drowsiness, dizziness, or light-headedness
- vivid dreams
- nervousness, anxiety, or difficulty sleeping
- unusual muscle stiffness or muscle twitching
- decreased sexual interest or function
- decreased appetite
- diarrhea or constipation
- sweating

Time Required for Drug to Take Effect: Some
patients may notice improved appetite or sleep within
the first few weeks, but full benefit may take from 4 to
8 weeks.

Symptoms of Overdose:
- extreme drowsiness or weakness
- seizures
- rapid heartbeat

Special Notes:

- Venlafaxine may interact with several other medicines commonly taken by older adults. To avoid potential interactions, show your doctor and pharmacist a complete list of all medicines, including nonprescription medicines, which you take regularly or on occasion.
- Never increase your dose without the advice of your doctor. Even small changes in dose may increase the risk of unwanted effects.
- Venlafaxine may cause an increase in blood pressure. Have your blood pressure checked regularly.
- Know which "target symptoms" (restlessness, worry, fear, or changes in sleep or appetite) you are being treated for and be prepared to tell your doctor if your target symptoms are improving, worsening, or unchanged.
- Do not discontinue without first talking with your doctor.
- Do not drink alcohol while taking this medication.

verapamil

Brand Names:

Calan (Searle)
Calan SR (Searle)
Isoptin (Knoll)

Isoptin SR (Knoll)
Verelan (Lederle)

Generic Available: yes

Type of Drug: cardiovascular (calcium channel blocker)

Used for: Treatment of angina, high blood pressure (hypertension), and abnormal heart rhythms (arrhythmias).

How This Medication Works: Inhibits smooth-muscle contraction and causes blood vessels to dilate.

Dosage Form and Strength:
- tablets (40 mg, 80 mg, 120 mg)
- sustained-release tablets (120 mg, 180 mg, 240 mg)
- sustained-release capsules (120 mg, 180 mg, 240 mg)

Storage:
- room temperature
- protected from humidity

Administration:
- Take verapamil at the same time every day.
- Swallow sustained-release tablets and capsules whole; do not crush or chew.
- Take sustained-release capsules or tablets with food or milk.

Precautions:
Do not use if:
- you have ever had an allergic reaction to verapamil or another calcium channel blocker such as amlodipine, diltiazem, or nifedipine.
Talk to your doctor if:
- you have heart disease, kidney disease, liver disease, or problems with circulation or your blood vessels.

- you are taking any other medications, especially carbamazepine, cyclosporin, or warfarin.

Side Effects:

Major:
- bleeding or bruising, especially in the gums
- skin rash, itching
- difficulty breathing
- slow heartbeat (less than 50 beats per minute)
- chest pressure or discomfort
- fainting
- swelling of ankles, feet, or lower legs

Minor:
- low blood pressure (light-headedness, dizziness)
- headache
- sexual dysfunction
- flushing
- drowsiness
- nausea, constipation
- tiredness

Time Required for Drug to Take Effect: Starts
to work within 2 hours. However, it takes at least 2 to 4 weeks to see the maximal response.

Symptoms of Overdose:

- nausea and vomiting
- weakness
- dizziness
- drowsiness
- confusion
- slurred speech
- heart palpitations
- loss of consciousness

Special Notes:
- Verapamil is not a cure, and you may have to take this medication for a long time.
- Changing positions slowly when sitting and/or standing up may help decrease dizziness caused by this medication. If light-headedness or dizziness occurs, it is important not to perform activities requiring mental alertness, such as driving a car or operating machinery.
- Check with your physician or pharmacist before using any over-the-counter medications.
- Ask your doctor to tell you the range for a safe heart rate, but generally it is important to call your physician if your heart rate falls below 50 beats per minute.
- Be careful to avoid becoming dehydrated or overheated. Avoid saunas and strenuous exercise in hot weather; avoid alcoholic beverages; and drink plenty of fluids.
- The active drug in the extended-release tablets is released through osmosis. Sometimes, the ghost of the tablet may show up in the stool and appear not to have been absorbed. However, the active ingredient will have been absorbed.

warfarin

Brand Name: Coumadin (DuPont)

Generic Available: no

Type of Drug: anticoagulant

Used for: Prevention of blood-clot formation.

How This Medication Works: Inhibits the clotting ability of the blood.

Dosage Form and Strength: tablets (1 mg, 2 mg, 2.5 mg, 5 mg, 7.5 mg, 10 mg)

Storage:
- room temperature
- tightly closed
- protected from light

Administration:
- Doses differ for each person.
- Usually taken in the evening.
- If you forget to take a dose, do not double the amount the next day; take the usual dose that your doctor has prescribed. Missing only one dose will not cause a clot to form. Missing more than one dose may cause problems; tell your doctor if you miss more than one dose. The dose required to keep a clot from forming is often very close to the dose that may cause bleeding; taking more than prescribed may cause bleeding.

Precautions:
Do not use if:
- you have had an allergic reaction to warfarin.

Talk to your doctor if:
- you have a stomach ulcer.
- you have ever had a stroke.
- you are taking any medication, especially allopurinol, amiodarone, anabolic steroids, chloral

hydrate, chloramphenicol, chlorpropamide, cimetidine, clofibrate, danazol, disulfiram, erythromycin, gemfibrozil, glucagon, influenza vaccine, isoniazid, ketoconazole, methimazole, methyldopa, methylphenidate, metronidazole, monoamine oxidase (MAO) inhibitors (such as phenelzine or tranylcypromine), nalidixic acid, phenylbutazone, propoxyphene, quinidine, quinine, salicylates, sulfamethoxazole, trimethoprim, sulfinpyrazone, sulfonamides, sulindac, tetracycline, thyroid hormones, azathioprine, barbiturates, birth control pills, carbamazepine, cholestyramine, colestipol, diuretics, estrogens, ethchlorvynol, griseofulvin, phenytoin, propylthiouracil, rifampin, sucralfate, vitamin K, adrenocorticosteroids (such as prednisone or dexamethasone), anticancer drugs, aspirin, diflunisal, dipyridamole, fenoprofen, ibuprofen, indomethacin, oxyphenbutazone, phenylbutazone, potassium, quinidine, quinine, salicylates, oral diabetes medications (such as glipizide, glyburide, or tolbutamide), and phenytoin.

Side Effects:

Major:

- severe back pain
- bleeding gums
- black, tarry stools or red blood in your stools
- blue or purple, painful toes
- unusual, frequent, or severe bruising
- chills or fever
- coughing up blood
- cuts or wounds that won't stop bleeding

- decreased alertness
- diarrhea
- blood in eyes
- headache (severe or persistent)
- joint pain or swelling
- heavy or unexpected menstrual bleeding
- nausea or vomiting
- nose bleeds
- paralysis or speech difficulty
- persistent sore throat
- stomach pain or bloating
- bloody, pink, or red tinged urine
- unusual tiredness, weakness, or unsteadiness
- yellow eyes or skin (jaundice)

Minor:
- loss of appetite
- gas or bloated stomach
- blurred vision
- hair loss

Time Required for Drug to Take Effect: Varies by patient, dose, and reason for therapy.

Symptoms of Overdose: See Major Side Effects.

Special Notes:
- While you are taking warfarin, your doctor will periodically monitor therapy with blood tests.
- It is important that all of your doctors be aware that you are taking warfarin.
- Check with your physician or pharmacist before using any over-the-counter medications.
- Changes in diet may affect the way warfarin works. Maintain a steady, well-balanced diet. Too

many leafy green vegetables on consecutive days may alter your bleeding time; you should eat the same weekly balance of vegetables.
- Do not drink alcohol while taking this medication.
- Tell the doctor or dentist you are taking warfarin if you are going to have any medical procedure or emergency treatment. You should wear some type of identification that says that you are on this medication in case an accident or injury occurs.
- Talk to your doctor about exercising.
- Do not change brand of this medication without checking with your doctor.
- You should never take more or less medication than is prescribed by the doctor.

zolpidem

Brand Name: Ambien (Searle)

Generic Available: no

Type of Drug: sedatives

Used for: Treatment of insomnia.

How This Medication Works: Reduces electrical activity in brain.

Dosage Form and Strength: tablets (5 mg, 10 mg)

Storage:
- room temperature
- tightly closed

Administration:
- Take on an empty stomach.
- Do not take more than prescribed amount.
- If you miss a dose, take the next when it is scheduled; do not double doses.

Precautions:
Do not use if:
- you have had an allergic reaction to zolpidem.

Talk to your doctor if:
- you are taking any other medications, especially chlorpromazine, imipramine, or other medications that may depress the central nervous system.
- you have liver disease or lung disease such as emphysema, asthma, or bronchitis.
- you feel you need to continue this medicine for more than 7 days.
- you have been told that you snore.

Side Effects:
Major:
- clumsiness
- confusion
- rash
- irritability
- hallucinations

Minor:
- abnormal dreams
- dizziness or double vision
- dry mouth
- diarrhea
- nausea or vomiting
- headache

Time Required for Drug to Take Effect:
Begins to work within 15 to 30 minutes.

Symptoms of Overdose:
- severe dizziness
- nausea and vomiting
- double vision

Special Notes:
- Do not drink alcohol while taking this medication.
- Use of zolpidem should be limited to 7 to 10 days.

Brand Names

Brand Name	**Generic Name**
Aceta with Codeine	codeine and acetaminophen combination
Adalat	nifedipine
Adalat CC	nifedipine
Adapin	doxepin
Advil	ibuprofen
Aerolate	theophylline
Aldactone	spironolactone
Aldomet	methyldopa
Aleve	naproxen sodium
Alupent	metaproterenol
Amacodone	hydrocodone and acetaminophen combination
Amaphen	butalbital, acetaminophen, and caffeine combination
Ambien	zolpidem
Amen	medroxyprogesterone
Amoxil	amoxicillin
Anaprox	naproxen sodium
Anexsia	hydrocodone and acetaminophen combination
Antivert	meclizine
Antrizine	meclizine
Apresoline	hydralazine
Aristocort	triamcinolone (topical)
Artane	trihexyphenidyl
Artane Sequels	trihexyphenidyl
Arthropan	salicylate salts (choline salicylate)
Atarax	hydroxyzine
Ativan	lorazepam
Atrovent	ipratropium
Augmentin	amoxicillin and clavulanic acid combination
Aventyl	nortriptyline
Axid Pulvules	nizatidine
Azmacort	triamcinolone acetonide (inhaler)

BRAND NAME	GENERIC NAME
Catapres	clonidine
Catapres-TTS	clonidine
Ceftin	cefuroxime
Cibacalcin	calcitonin
Cibalith-S	lithium
Cipro	ciprofloxacin
Claritin	loratadine
Climara	estradiol
Clozaril	clozapine
Co-Gesic	hydrocodone and acetaminophen combination
Cogentin	benztropine
Cognex	tacrine
Compazine	prochlorperazine
Condrin-LA	phenylpropanolamine and chlorpheniramine combination
Congess Sr	pseudoephedrine and guaifenesin combination
Congestac Caplets	pseudoephedrine and guaifenesin combination
Constant-T	theophylline
Contac 12-Hour	phenylpropanolamine and chlorpheniramine combination
Cordarone	amiodarone
Cotrim	sulfamethoxazole and trimethoprim combination
Coumadin	warfarin
Cozaar	losartan
Curretab	medroxyprogesterone
Cycrin	medroxyprogesterone
Cytotec	misoprostol
Dalmane	flurazepam
Dantrium	dantrolene
Darvocet-N100	propoxyphene napsylate and acetaminophen combination
Darvocet-N50	propoxyphene napsylate and acetaminophen combination
Daypro	oxaprozin
Dazamide	acetazolamide
Decadron	dexamethasone

BRAND NAME	GENERIC NAME
Deconsal II	pseudoephedrine and guaifenesin combination
Deltasone	prednisone
Demerol	meperidine
Depakene	valproic acid
Depakote	valproic acid
Depakote Sprinkle	valproic acid
Desyrel	trazodone
Dexone	dexamethasone
Di-Spaz	dicyclomine
DiaBeta	glyburide
Diamox	acetazolamide
Dilacor XR	diltiazem
Dilantin	phenytoin
Dilatrate-SR	isosorbide dinitrate
Dipentum	olsalazine
Disalcid	salsalate
Ditropan	oxybutynin
Dizmiss	meclizine
Dolacet	hydrocodone and acetaminophen combination
Dopar	levodopa
Doryx	doxycycline
Drize	phenylpropanolamine and chlorpheniramine combination
Dura-Vent/A	phenylpropanolamine and chlorpheniramine combination
Duradyne DHC	hydrocodone and acetaminophen combination
Duragesic-100	fentanyl
Duragesic-25	fentanyl
Duragesic-50	fentanyl
Duragesic-75	fentanyl
Duvoid	bethanechol
Dyazide	triamterene and hydrochlorothiazide combination
E-Mycin	erythromycin
Effexor	venlafaxine
Elavil	amitriptyline
Eldepryl	selegiline

BRAND NAME	GENERIC NAME
Elixophyllin	theophylline
Elixophyllin SR	theophylline
Endep	amitriptyline
Endolor	butalbital, acetaminophen, and caffeine combination
Enovil	amitriptyline
Entex PSE	pseudoephedrine and guaifenesin combination
Epitol	carbamazepine
Ery-Tab	erythromycin
Eryc	erythromycin
Esgic	butalbital, acetaminophen, and caffeine combination
Esidrix	hydrochlorothiazide
Eskalith	lithium
Estraderm	estradiol
Fedahist Expectorant Syrup	pseudoephedrine and guaifenesin combination
Feldene	piroxicam
Feosol	ferrous sulfate
Fer-In-Sol Syrup	ferrous sulfate
Fero-Gradumet	ferrous sulfate
Fioricet	butalbital, acetaminophen, and caffeine combination
Flagyl	metronidazole
Flexeril	cyclobenzaprine
Flumadine	rimantadine
Folvite	folic acid
Fosamax	alendronate
Fulvicin P/G	griseofulvin
Fulvicin U/F	griseofulvin
Furadantin	nitrofurantoin
Gastrocrom	cromolyn
Glucophage	metformin
Glucotrol	glipizide
Glucotrol XL	glipizide
Glynase Prestab	glyburide
Grifulvin V	griseofulvin
Gris-PEG	griseofulvin
Grisactin Ultra	griseofulvin

BRAND NAME	GENERIC NAME
GuaiCough PE	pseudoephedrine and guaifenesin combination
Guaifed	pseudoephedrine and guaifenesin combination
Guaifed Syrup	pseudoephedrine and guaifenesin combination
Guaifed-PD	pseudoephedrine and guaifenesin combination
GuaiMax-D	pseudoephedrine and guaifenesin combination
Guaitab	pseudoephedrine and guaifenesin combination
Guaituss PE Syrup	pseudoephedrine and guaifenesin combination
Habitrol	nicotine
Halcion	triazolam
Haldol	haloperidol
Halotussin PE	pseudoephedrine and guaifenesin combination
Haltran	ibuprofen
Histalet X	pseudoephedrine and guaifenesin combination
Humalog	insulin lispro
Humulin	insulin
Hy-Phen	hydrocodone and acetaminophen combination
HydroDiuril	hydrochlorothiazide
Hydrogesic	hydrocodone and acetaminophen combination
Iletin	insulin
Imdur	isosorbide mononitrate
Inderal	propranolol
Inderal LA	propranolol
Indocin	indomethacin
Indocin CR	indomethacin
Intal	cromolyn
ISMO	isosorbide mononitrate
Isoptin	verapamil
Isoptin SR	verapamil
Isordil	isosorbide dinitrate

BRAND NAME	GENERIC NAME
Lupron Depot	leuprolide
Macrobid	nitrofurantoin
Macrodantin	nitrofurantoin
Maxolon	metoclopramide
Maxzide	triamterene and hydrochloro-thiazide combination
Medigesic	butalbital, acetaminophen, and caffeine combination
Medrol	methylprednisolone
Mellaril	thioridazine
Meni-D	meclizine
Metaprel	metaproterenol
Meticorten	prednisone
Mevacor	lovastatin
Miacalcin	calcitonin
Micronase	glyburide
Minipress	prazosin
Minitran	nitroglycerin
Mol-Iron	ferrous sulfate
Monoket	isosorbide mononitrate
Motrin	ibuprofen
MS Contin	morphine
MSIR	morphine
Mycelex	clotrimazole
Mykrox	metolazone
Mysoline	primidone
Naprelan	naproxen
Naprosyn	naproxen
Nasalcrom	cromolyn
Navane	thiothixene
Neurontin	gabapentin
Nicoderm	nicotine
Nicotrol	nicotine
Nitro-Bid Ointment	nitroglycerin
Nitro-Dur	nitroglycerin
NitroBid Plateau caps	nitroglycerin
Nitrodisc	nitroglycerin
Nitrol Ointment	nitroglycerin
Nitrolingual Spray	nitroglycerin
Nitrong	nitroglycerin

BRAND NAME	GENERIC NAME
Nitrostat	nitroglycerin
Nizoral	ketoconazole
Noctec	chloral hydrate
Nolvadex	tamoxifen
Normodyne	labetalol
Norvasc	amlodipine
Novolin	insulin
Nuprin	ibuprofen
Omnipen	ampicillin
Oragest TD	phenylpropanolamine and chlorpheniramine combination
Oramorph SR	morphine
Orasone	prednisone
Oretic	hydrochlorothiazide
Ornade	phenylpropanolamine and chlorpheniramine combination
OxyContin	oxycodone
Pamelor	nortriptyline
Paxil	paroxetine
PCE Dispertab	erythromycin
Pepcid	famotidine
Percocet	oxycodone and acetaminophen combination
Periactin	cyproheptadine
Parlodel	bromocriptine
Permax	pergolide
Persantine	dipyridamole
Phenameth	promethazine
Phenaphen-650 with Codeine	codeine and acetaminophen combination
Phenaphen with Codeine	codeine and acetaminophen combination
Phenergan	promethazine
Phenergan Fortis	promethazine
Phenergan Plain	promethazine
Phenergan with Codeine	promethazine and codeine combination
Pherazine with Codeine	promethazine and codeine combination

BRAND NAME	GENERIC NAME
Septra DS	sulfamethoxazole and trimethoprim combination
Serax	oxazepam
Serevent	salmeterol
Serzone	nefazodone
Sinemet	levodopa and carbidopa combination
Sinemet CR	levodopa and carbidopa combination
Sinequan	doxepin
Sinufed Timecelles	pseudoephedrine and guaifenesin combination
Slo-bid Gyrocaps	theophylline
Slo-Phyllin	theophylline
Slo-Phyllin Gyrocaps	theophylline
Soma	carisoprodol
Soma Compound	carisoprodol and aspirin combination
Soma Compound with Codeine	carisoprodol, aspirin, and codeine combination
Sorbitrate	isosorbide dinitrate
Sporanox	itraconazole
Stelazine	trifluoperazine
Sustaire	theophylline
Symadine	amantadine
Symmetrel	amantadine
Synthroid	levothyroxine
T-Phyl	theophylline
Tagamet	cimetidine
Talwin	pentazocine
Tegretol	carbamazepine
Tencon	butalbital and acetaminophen combination
Tenormin	atenolol
Theo-24	theophylline
Theo-Dur	theophylline
Theo-Sav	theophylline
Theobid Duracaps	theophylline
Theobid Jr. Duratuss	theophylline
Theoclear LA	theophylline

BRAND NAME	GENERIC NAME
Theolair	theophylline
Theolair-SR	theophylline
Theospan-SR	theophylline
Theovent	theophylline
Theox	theophylline
Thorazine	chlorpromazine
Tiazac	diltiazem
Ticlid	ticlopidine
Timoptic	timolol
Tofranil	imipramine
Tofranil-PM	imipramine
Toprol XL	metoprolol
Toradol	ketorolac
Totacillin	ampicillin
Trandate	labetalol
Transderm-Nitro	nitroglycerin
Triaprin	butalbital and acetaminophen combination
Trilafon	perphenazine
Trilisate	salicylate salts (choline magnesium trisalicylate)
Trimox	amoxicillin
Triphenyl	phenylpropanolamine and chlorpheniramine combination
Tuss-LA	pseudoephedrine and guaifenesin combination
Ty-tabs	codeine and acetaminophen combination
Tylenol with Codeine	codeine and acetaminophen combination
Tylox	oxycodone and acetaminophen combination
Ultram	tramadol
Uniphyl	theophylline
Urecholine	bethanechol
V-Dec-M	pseudoephedrine and guaifenesin combination
Valisone	betamethasone valerate
Valium	diazepam
Valrelease	diazepam

BRAND NAME	GENERIC NAME
Vanceril	beclomethasone dipropionate
Vasotec	enalapril
Ventolin	albuterol
Verelan	verapamil
Versacaps	pseudoephedrine and guaifenesin combination
Vibramycin	doxycycline
Vibra-tabs	doxycycline
Vicodin	hydrocodone and acetaminophen combination
Vicodin ES	hydrocodone and acetaminophen combination
Vistaril	hydroxyzine
Vivelle	estradiol
Voltaren	diclofenac
Wellbutrin	bupropion
Wymox	amoxicillin
Xanax	alprazolam
Zantac	ranitidine
Zaroxolyn	metolazone
Zephrex	pseudoephedrine and guaifenesin combination
Zephrex-LA	pseudoephedrine and guaifenesin combination
Zestril	lisinopril
Zithromax	azithromycin
Zocor	simvastatin
Zoloft	sertraline
Zovirax	acyclovir
Zydone	hydrocodone and acetaminophen combination
Zyloprim	allopurinol

Canadian Brand Names

Brand Name (Manufacturer)	Generic Name
Acet-Am (Organon)	theophylline
Acetazolam(ICN)	acetazolamide
Alloprin (ICN)	allopurinol
Amersol (Horner)	ibuprofen
Ampicin (Bristol)	ampicillin
Ampilean (Organon)	ampicillin
Apo-Acetazolamide (Apotex)	acetazolamide
Apo-Allopurinol (Apotex)	allopurinol
Apo-Amitriptyline (Apotex)	amitriptyline
Apo-Amoxi (Apotex)	amoxicillin
Apo-Ampi (Apotex)	ampicillin
Apo-Atenolol (Apotex)	atenolol
Apo-Benztropine (Apotex)	benztropine
Apo-Carbamazepine (Apotex)	carbamazepine
Apo-Cephalex (Apotex)	cephalexin
Apo-Diazapam (Apotex)	diazepam
Apo-Dipyridamole (Apotex)	dipyridamole
Apo-Doxy (Apotex)	doxycycline
Apo-Ferrous Sulfate (Apotex)	ferrous sulfate
Apo-Flurazepam (Apotex)	flurazepam
Apo-Folic (Apotex)	folic acid
Apo-Furosemide (Apotex)	furosemide
Apo-Hydro (Apotex)	hydrochlorothiazide
Apo-Hydroxyzine (Apotex)	hydroxyzine
Apo-Imipramine (Apotex)	imipramine
Apo-Lorazepam (Apotex)	lorazepam
Apo-metoprolol (Apotex)	metoprolol
Apo-Naproxen (Apotex)	naproxen
Apo-Nifed (Apotex)	nifedipine
Apo-Nitrofurantoin Apotex)	nitrofurantoin
Apo-Oxazepam (Apotex)	oxazepam
Apo-Perphenazine (Apotex)	perphenazine
Apo-Prednisone (Apotex)	prednisone
Apo-Primidone (Apotex)	primidone
Apo-Propranolol (Apotex)PMS	propranolol
Apo-Quinidine (Apotex)	quinidine

BRAND NAME (MANUFACTURER)	GENERIC NAME
Apo-Timol (Apotex)	timolol
Apo-Trihex (Apotex)	trihexyphenidyl
Apo-Verap (Apotex)	verapamil
Becloforte (Glaxo)	beclomethasone dipropionate (inhaler)
Bentylol (Merrell)	dicyclomine
Betaloc (Astra)	metoprolol
Betalox (Astra)	metoprolol
Biquin Durules (Astra)	quinidine
Bonamine (Pfizer)	meclizine
C.E.S. (Allergan)	estrogens, conjugated
Canesten (Miles)	clotrimazole
Carbolith (ICN)	lithium
Ceporex (Glaxo)	cephalexin
Chlorpromanyl (Technilab)	chlorpromazine
Clavulin (Beecham)	amoxicillin and clavulanic acid
Congest (Trianon Laboratories)	estrogens, conjugated
Coronex (Ayerst)	isosorbide dinitrate
Deronil (Schering)	dexamethasone
Detensol (Desbergers)	propranolol
Diuchlor H (Medic)	hydrochlorothiazide
Dopamet (ICN)	methyldopa
Eltroxin (Glaxo)	levothyroxine
Emex (Beecham)	metoclopramide
Epimorph (Ayerst)	morphine
Erythromid (Abbott)	erythromycin
Euglucon (Boehringer Ingelheim)	glyburide
Fivent (Fisons)	cromolyn
Histanil (Pharmascience)	promethazine
Impril (ICN)	imipramine
Indocid (MSD)	indomethacin
Insulin-Toronto (Connaught NovoNordisk)	insulin
Isotamine (ICN)	isoniazide
Largactid (Rhone-Poulenc)	chlorpromazine
Lenoltec with Codeine (Technilab)	codeine and acetaminophen
Levate (ICN)	amitriptyline
Lithizine (Maney)	lithium

BRAND NAME (MANUFACTURER)	GENERIC NAME
Lotriderm (Schering)	clotrimazole and beta-methasone
M.O.S. (ICN)	morphine
M.O.S.-S.R. (ICN)	morphine
Maxeran (Nordic)	metoclopramide
Mazepine (ICN)	carbamazepine
Medilium (Medic)	chlordiazepoxide
Multipax (Rhone-Poulenc Rorer)	hydroxyzine
Myclo (Boehringer Ingelheim)	clotrimazole
Naxen (SynCare)	naproxen
Neo-Codema (Neolab)	hydrochlorothiazide
Neo-Metric (Neolab)	metronidazole
Nephronex (Cortunon)	nitrofurantoin
Novamoxin (Novopharm)	amoxicillin
Novo-Atenol (Novopharm)	atenolol
Novo-Carbamaz (Novopharm)	carbamazepine
Novo-Chlorhydrate (Novopharm)	chloral hydrate
Novo-Colchicine (Novopharm)	colchicine
Novo-Digoxin (Novopharm)	digoxin
Novo-Doxylin (Novopharm)	doxycycline
Novo-Folacid (Novopharm)	folic acid
Novo-Hydroxyzin (Novopharm)	hydroxyzine
Novo-Hylazin (Novopharm)	hydralazine
Novo-Lorazem (Novopharm)	lorazepam
Novo-Metoprol (Novopharm)	metoprolol
Novo-Naprox (Novopharm)	naproxen
Novo-Nifedin (Novopharm)	nifedipine
Novo-Pranol (Novopharm)	propranolol
Novo-Quinidin (Novopharm)	quinidine
Novo-Salmol (Novopharm)	albuterol
Novo-Veramil (Novopharm)	verapamil
Novocimetine (Novopharm)	cimetidine
Novodipam (Novopharm)	diazepam
Novoferrosulfa (Novopharm)	ferrous sulfate
Novoflupam (Novopharm)	flurazepam
Novofuran (Novopharm)	nitrofurantoin
Novohexidyl (Novopharm)	trihexyphenidyl
Novohydrazide (Novopharm)	hydrochlorothiazide
Novolexin (Novopharm)	cephalexin

BRAND NAME (MANUFACTURER)	GENERIC NAME
Novolin-Toronto (Connaught NovoNordisk)	insulin
Novomedopa (Novopharm)	methyldopa
Novomethacin (Novopharm)	indomethacin
Novonaprox (Novopharm)	naproxen
Novonidazole (Novopharm)	metronidazole
Novopoxide (Novopharm)	chlordiazepoxide
Novopramine (Novopharm)	imipramine
Novoprofen (Novopharm)	ibuprofen
Novopropoxyn (Novopharm)	propoxyohene
Novopurol (Novopharm)	allopurinol
Novoridazine (Novopharm)	thioridazine
Novosemide (Novopharm)	furosemide
Novosorbide(Novopharm)	isosorbide dinitrate
Novospiroton (Novopharm)	spironolactone
Novotriamzide (Novopharm)	triamterene and hydro-chlorothiazide
Novotrimel (Novopharm)	sulfamethoxizole and trimethoprim
Novotriptyn (Novopharm)	amitriptyline
Nu-Amoxi (Nu-Pharm)	amoxicillin
Nu-Cephalex (Nu-Pharm)	cephalexin
Nu-Loraz (Nu-Pharm)	lorazepam
Nu-Metop (Nu-Pharm)	metoprolol
Nu-Naprox (Nu-Pharm)	naproxen
Nu-Nifed (Nu-Pharm)	nifedipine
Nu-Verap (Nu-Pharm)	verapamil
Oxycocet (Technilab)	oxycodone and aceta-minophen
Penbritin (Ayerst)	ampicillin
Peptol (Horner)	cimetidine
Peridol (Technilab)	haloperidol
Pertrofrane (Geigy)	desipramine
Phenazo (ICN)	phenazopyridine
PMS Benztropine (Pharmascience)	benztropine
PMS Perphenazine (Pharmascience)	perphenazine
PMS Primidone (Pharmascience)	primidone
PMS Prochlorperazine (Pharmascience)	prochlorperazine
PMS-Isoniazid (Pharmascience)	isoniazide
PMS Propranolol (Pharmascience)	propranolol

BRAND NAME (MANUFACTURER)	GENERIC NAME
Prepulsid (Janssen)	cisapride
Purinol (Horner)	allopurinol
Quinate (Rougler)	quinidine
Renedil (Hoechst)	felodipine
Rofact (ICN)	rifampin
Roubac (Rougier)	sulfamethoxizole and trimethoprim
Rounox with Codeine (Rougier)	codeine and acetaminophen
Rynacrom (Fisons)	cromolyn
Salazopyrin (Pharmacia)	sulfasalazine
Sertan (Pharmascience)	primidone
Solazine (Horner)	trifluperazine
Solium (Horner)	chlordiazepoxide
Som-Pam (ICN)	flurazepam
Somnol (Horner)	flurazepam
Statex (Pharmascience)	morphine
Stemetil (May & Baker)	prochlorperazine
Stemetil (Rhone-Poulenc Rorer)	prochlorperazine
Sulcrate (Technilab)	sucralfate
Tamofen (Rhone-Poulenc Rorer)	tamoxifen
Tamone (Adria)	tamoxifen
Triadapin (Fisons)	doxepin
Uritol (Horner)	furosemide
Vivol (Horner)	diazepam
Warfilone (Frosst)	warfarin
Winpred (ICN)	prednisone
Zapex (Riva)	oxazepam

General Index